# TENDON & LIGAMENT HEALING

## A NEW APPROACH TO SPORTS AND OVERUSE INJURY

### WILLIAM WEINTRAUB

Paradigm Publications

Brookline Massachusetts and Taos New Mexico

2 0 0 3

# Tendon and Ligament Healing
## A New Approach to Sports and Overuse Injury
### *Second revised and expanded edition*

©2003 William Weintraub
ISBN 0-912111-73-9

Body Mind Centering® is a registered service mark and BMCSM is a service mark of Bonnie Bainbridge Cohen

Library of Congress Cataloging-in-Publication information for the first edition is as follows:

Library of Congress Cataloging-in-Publication Information:
Weintraub, William, 1945-
  Tendon and ligament healing : a new approach through manual therapy /
William Weintraub.
    p. cm.
*Sponsored by the Society for the Study of Native Arts and Sciences" T.p. verso.
  Includes bibliographical references.
    ISBN 1-55643-283-6
1. Tendons Wounds and injuries-Physical therapy. 2. Ligaments-Wounds and
injuries-Physical therapy. 3. Manipulation (Therapeutics) I. Society for the Study
of Native Arts and Sciences. II. Title.
[DNLM: 1. Tendon injuries-rehabilitation. 2. Ligaments-Injuries. 3.
Manipulation, Orthopedic. 4. Chronic Disease-rehabilitation. WE 600 W424t
1998]
RC688.245  1999
617.4'74044-dc21
DNLM/DLC
For Library of Congress                                              98-17726
                                                                          CIP

Cover design by Herb Rich III
Cover photograph by Don Jacot
Text drawings and photographs by Don Jacot
Cartoons by Tamara Herendeen and Diane Sherman
Published by Paradigm Publications
Brookline, Massachusetts and Taos, New Mexico
www.paradigm-pubs.com

# TABLE OF CONTENTS

Bill Weintraub, M.S. is at the same time an excellent therapist and a researcher who has produced a very valuable, highly interesting work in the area of tendon and ligament treatment. This book is clear and comprehensive. It is a great pleasure for me to write this preface because it is due to people like him that manual therapy gains increased acceptance in the medical world.

A therapist who is effective in relieving people's suffering deserves our encouragement and gratitude for providing help to other practitioners in the areas of treatment and research; it's so important to share our experience with others.

Modern physiology teaches us that the finest and most sensitive proprioceptors are located in tendons and ligaments. Relieving stress on the mechanoreceptors located in these structures produces specific effects through local feedback systems, permitting the release of joint and muscle problems. These nerve receptors are also part of a larger feedback loop which can provide a general benefit to the body through spinal, cerebellar, and brain stimulation. Weintraub's thorough, precise treatment methods for the tendon or ligament stimulate neural input which emanates from that local structure, and is received centrally by the organism; this causes a favorable reciprocal effect on the localized injury area from the Central Nervous System.

The structural and neural activity described above also allows beneficial repatterning of larger body functions such as orchestration of complex movements, permitting the patient to feel better in his or her life. In these ways the health of tendons and ligaments plays a role in both physical and emotional homeostasis. The soundly-based treatment options presented in this book for recovery from chronic injury bring benefits on multiple levels.

Effective treatment of these injuries is a crucial and challenging area of health care, welcoming Bill Weintraub's promising new approach here. This is why his work with osteopathic and related therapies is such an important contribution in this field.

Jean-Pierre Barral, D.O.

# PREFACE

It gives me pleasure to write this preface to Tendon and Ligament Healing by Bill Weintraub. I believe this is an important publication because of the skills, light, and optimism it brings to the problem of chronic tendon/ligament injuries. The book will be helpful to anyone engaged in therapy of joints and soft tissue, especially of the tendon and ligament variety, or to anyone who has sustained this type of injury and has not made satisfactory recovery. It will hold strong interest for the person who is drawn to a health care model based on the self-corrective powers of the body.

Weintraub crafted his own professional training instead of following the traditional and highly organized schools of medicine or physiotherapy, where treatment modalities are quite standardized. He escaped a certain pessimism so often inherent in the standard treatment of chronic tendon and ligament injuries. The underpinnings of his training were experiential in nature involving sports, yoga and dance. He had already embodied a sense of optimum form and function within his own body before he began his more formal study of anatomy and pathology. As he entered into the healing arts he studied with people who themselves came from personal experience and nontraditional sources. He was influenced by acupressure and Chinese theory of wholeness, and studied at length with innovative osteopaths who were continuing to expand possibilities based on deeper understanding of anatomy and touch.

With this training and background Weintraub was not limited to the traditional teachings of chronic tissue injury. He experientially learned the micro-anatomy of ligaments and tendons through touch;

and he has developed a creative approach, using in-depth manual skills to aid chronic injury and dysfunction. The method is firmly grounded in osteopathic tradition. In addition, realizing the importance of the whole person, he went full circle to involve the patient in their own healing process. This book is full of useful suggestions. His combined approach has been successful and has led to an optimistic attitude for a person's recovery, which itself aids the process.

The personal application of his own methods and beliefs help validate what he presents in this book. When Weintraub sustained a chronic tendon injury from excessive weight lifting, he applied his methodology to his own injury and recovered, despite a negative prognosis given by several orthopedists. He actualized the famous axiom, "physician heal thyself."

Bill Weintraub is to be congratulated for his insights, optimism and a fresh approach to chronic tendon and ligament problems. His understanding of how to specifically benefit the micro-anatomy through touch, and his inclusion of the whole person in healing, offer new possibilities for therapists and patients alike when dealing with these difficult problems. This is a timely book.

Fritz Frederick Smith, M.D.

# ACKNOWLEDGEMENTS

Thanks to all my teachers, patients, and students for the development of my work. Thanks to my father, Louis Weintraub. To my overall mentor, Lew Colburn. To Neala Haze, partner through many phases. I've been fortunate to have so much help with this book: special thanks to Shierry Nicholsen for wise guidance, Don Jacot for illustrations and photos, Bob Felt and Martha Fielding for publishing, and to David Lippincott, Betsy Partridge, Paul Boudakian, Edith Gladstone, Mary Ruth Hammond, Alan Leveton, Cathy Adachi, Harold McCoy, Diane Sherman, Winnie Ganshaw, and Paula Koepke.

# NOTE TO THE GENERAL READER
## (NON-CLINICIANS)

I have aimed to make all portions of this book as clear as possible. Non-clinical readers should find all material easily accessible, with the possible exception of some parts of Chapter 2 (21-45), Chapter 3 (56-79), and Chapter 5. The drawings and photos in those sections will be very useful. You find an overview of the whole topic and map of the book in Chapter 1.

# ABOUT SPORTS INJURY

Sports-related damage to ligaments—like ankle sprains and jumper's knee, and tendon problems such as tennis elbow and Achilles tendinitis—are among the most frequent, chronic, and stubborn of all injuries. More than half of this book's case accounts illustrate hands-on therapy for people with sports injuries.

The greater emphasis now placed on physical activity and athletic performance is causing a rise in tendon and ligament injury. Up to 75 percent of all tendon ruptures are sports related. An increase in time and intensity of exercise and training has led to more frequent overuse problems for ligaments and tendons, accounting for up to 50 percent of all sports injury. Overuse damage results from endurance activity such as running or swimming as well as from repetitive activity using skill, technique, and power such as basketball, tennis, and ballet.

A view of the injury and healing process gives athletes, trainers, coaches, and fitness participants a sense of risk factors and preventive strategies. The sports section in Chapter 6 draws on recent research to present self-help guidelines for recovery, return to sports after injury, and exercise strategy.

This book presents the author's hands-on (manual) therapy model for tendon and ligament treatment. The reader will see its potential benefits for sports injuries.

# CHAPTER 1

# OVERVIEW

This book responds to a major challenge in the health care field. A high incidence of serious, chronic tendon and ligament injury causes substantial disability. The most widely used treatments often have unsuccessful results. And when seriously damaged, tendons and ligaments are not among the body parts more amenable to healing. I have made it a strong priority to find an effective method for reversing these sports and overuse injuries. The standard medical view is that non-surgical treatment has almost no chance of success once the injury has become chronic. In many cases surgery is only partially satisfactory or (in the long term) not at all.

In 29 years of practicing structural/osteopathic hands-on therapy I have done considerable work with seriously damaged tendons and ligaments and have developed a therapeutic model for treating these injuries, with beneficial results that would be considered highly improbable by conventional medicine. My approach offers people in chronic cases who have exhausted the standard physiotherapy and are facing surgery a viable option for recovery. The story of the dancer, Julia L., on the next page, is a capsule picture of this strategy.

Through a view of this innovative treatment approach and recent scientific research findings, the book explores the active nature and treatment of an often overlooked area (tendons and ligaments). It brings to light a basic bodily healing response, which can be important for strong self-maintenance and tissue healing of any part of the body.

The research points to surprisingly dynamic yet little-known properties of tendons/ ligaments that have highly favorable implications for their recovery potential.

The book's focus on manual (hands-on) therapy for athletic and workplace injury illustrates possibilities beyond the standard medical model for a creative approach to health care based on the body as a dynamic, responsive organism. Adaptability of the body is an essential principle, emerging from my clinical work and long-term exploration of health and physical awareness.

Clear, active perception is a key skill for a clinician. My therapy model combines this with well-trained technical/anatomical precision to apply its manual techniques for the body structure. Two in-depth case accounts and 15 additional cases in Chapter 4 directly illustrate this approach, along with the following brief account featuring the obstacles and therapy process of a chronic tendon injury.

Julia L. is a lifelong dancer who was very discouraged when she initially consulted me for a persistent problem with her right knee. A tall woman of forty-two, and now co-chair of a university dance department, she had stopped her workouts and was unable to demonstrate for her classes. Fifteen months earlier, when starting to dance after prolonged sitting on the floor of a cold studio, she noticed pain and stiffness of her posterior lateral knee that became a constant aching and burning sensation. This worsened and continued despite various medications, physiotherapy, chiropractic, and periods of rest. While bearing any weight on her knee, she was unable to bend it without weakness and a lot of pain. She was quite disconsolate, as she had been forced to reduce her teaching schedule and worried about her future in the profession to which she was very devoted.

An MRI scan revealed a substantial tear of the biceps femoris (lateral hamstring) tendon behind the knee joint. Four months after the initial injury two orthopedic surgeons felt there was no longer a realistic hope of recovery with conservative care. They proposed surgical repair of the tendon, which Julia was reluctant to undergo.

Julia agreed to my initial suggestion of three weekly treatments
to see if the structural/osteopathic
therapy I practice could help her
injury. I found significant swelling
of her posterior knee, along with
adhesion, weakness, "stringiness,"
and a twisted alignment pattern of
the tendon fibers as well as a palpable divot in the tendon where it
had been torn. I used gentle techniques to specifically free, align,
and tone the tendon fibers, as well
as free restrictions of her lower
spine and lower abdominal viscera.
Julia was cooperative in maintaining reduced activity levels and a
moderate exercise program. We
both noticed that gradually her
range and ease of knee joint mobility was increasing, swelling and
inflammation was reduced, and
pain was subsiding.

**Biceps Femoris Muscle**

**Outer Hamstring Tendon**

**Head of Fibula**

**Figure 1**
Posterior view of the right biceps
femoris (lateral hamstring) muscle
and its tendon at the knee.

After four weeks the frequency of treatments was reduced to two-
and then three-week intervals. I continued to treat restrictions of her
calf muscles and fascias, damage to the neighboring popliteal tendon,
and a stubborn fixation of the ankle joint and cuboid bone in her right
foot. After ten weeks she could climb a flight of stairs without pain and
comfortably walk one mile with moderate hills. She was optimistic
enough to be choreographing a piece in which she hoped to dance.
With continued manual therapy techniques the tendon fibers had been
realigned, their tone strengthened, adhesions almost eliminated, and
the defect in the tendon was filling in well.

At sessions three and then five months from starting therapy Julia could extend her knee completely and flex it to 110° and then 135° comfortably with weight-bearing (within 5° of normal). She was demonstrating for her classes with progressive ease and increasing her workouts. I found that the torn part of the tendon was very close to being intact and that the texture of the whole tendon was more resilient, "bouncy," with almost no laxity. Treatments went to one-month intervals, and after four of these Julia received two orthopedic evaluations of her knee as being normal. At that time she was very relieved and happy to resume a full teaching and workout schedule. She continued to feel quite well the following year.

Julia's story is very hopeful considering the extent and duration of her tendon injury. Hers was one of the high proportion of seriously damaged tendons and ligaments that become chronic. She had availed herself of the standard medical (and some nonmedical) treatments with the exception of surgery, about which she was hesitant in part because of uncertainty about its outcome. Julia had no major health problems preventing recovery and was quite cooperative through the course of treatment; these are important factors for the success of my therapy in the case of a stubborn condition.

This account gives a picture of strategies that reflect basic principles of structural health care, which have become clear through years in this field. These include the importance of precise anatomical focus and capacity to work with subtle changes of structure. Another essential principle is illustrated by my combining detailed, specific treatment of the small fibers and tissues of the local tendon injury area with an overall approach to improving larger body patterns and tensions. Therapeutic techniques for Julia's spine, muscles, fascias, visceral structures, and other joints helped to normalize the forces connected to the injury zone and promote its recovery. Progression of her case emphasizes the basic principle of responsiveness and capacity for self-correction of body tissues when given proper conditions.

Including its elements that are instructional for therapists, the book's primary theme is an informational source and guide that is both useful and provocative. This can shed light on the role of the therapist, self-help with injury, and sports/movement training. It addresses the question of what are realistic expectations for the function, health, and in-depth treatment of ligaments and tendons.

## A Manual Therapy Model—A New Approach

The primary techniques I used in Julia's case (and in all of my practice) are the osteopathic methods of Strain-Counterstrain, cranial and visceral osteopathy, and Fascial Release, as well as Body-Mind Centering, Joint Gliding, and specific tendon and ligament work. Also utilized are techniques from Zero Balancing, and from acupressure therapy, which was my initial training and licensing. All these methods individually and sometimes in combination have valuable aspects for treatment of tendons/ligaments, which will be discussed in later sections. I first worked with large numbers of these injuries in the mid-1970s when much of my practice in New York City consisted of dancers. Since then it has been a full-time practice involving all the major areas of structural health. These include: lower back and other spinal problems in the cervical area, visceral restrictions, nerve impingements, the cranial area, and peripheral joints such as the shoulder and ankle.

What actual changes are vital in the ligament or tendon tissue and related body systems in the healing process? Some are seen in Julia's recovery (e.g., reduction of adhesions) and there are a number of others that will be illustrated. The book relates these shifts of structure and function in healing to the therapy method(s) I use to promote the change.

The role of hands-on therapy in the conventional health care system is still very limited. In a system involving steep costs for highly technological and hospital-based interventions, incorporating the option of a noninvasive, effective treatment could be attractive.

My manual therapy model for treating these injuries consists of:

1. The osteopathic and other structural therapies that have been mentioned.

2. The way that I combine these methods and the specific usages to which they are directed.

3. The skills and aptitudes necessary for effective application of the techniques. This includes certain perceptual skills and thorough knowledge of anatomy and kinesiology.

This model I've developed represents a new approach to serious, chronic tendon and ligament injuries for a number of reasons:

- In the standard medical system in which most patients in this society are treated, manual therapy in any form is not an accepted strategy for reversing and healing major damage to tendons/ligaments once their condition has become chronic. While many physiotherapists train beyond the standard approach, conventional theory and practice mostly dictates that surgery is the only method with a realistic chance of success in this situation.

- Most of the therapy techniques in the model are innovative and not well known, and require thorough technical training for success with serious injuries.

- Application of these techniques is done in some original ways.

- The means by which I combine the methods is uncommon.

- Certain skills and aptitudes used to apply the clinical techniques (e.g., fine perception to detect subtle changes of structure and larger body patterns) are unusual; this is particularly the case in relation to applying these abilities to systematic, structurally accurate treatment of tendons and ligaments.

- There is a level of very specific, anatomically precise, in-depth, and inventive manual work with the often fragile intricacies of the ligament or tendon microstructure. These include particular strategies I use for aligning the small tendon fibers and their bundles, restoring their tone and reversing laxity, and working with the electrical activity of the tissues.

These features of my therapeutic model indicate its new approach for this type of injury. It is not expected that most practitioners use every element of the model, but that all may find important areas for exploration and focus.

Certain factors are positive or negative indicators for potential success in the application of my therapy in cases of serious injury. To present the positive side, an important favorable indicator is the patient's cooperation with recommendations for exercise and for reduced activity to avoid aggravation. Julia L., whose tendon treatment was mentioned earlier, is a good example of this. Also helpful are adequate nutrition and general health including absence of systemic disturbance of the connective tissue. The presence of certain negative factors (e.g., continued overuse or a connective tissue disorder) would greatly reduce the likelihood of full recovery. When the injury is severe it is vital for a successful outcome that the patient wants to recover.

There are benefits in skilled exercise and postural therapy, nutritional therapy including dietary supplements, and strategies for stress reduction. All these can be beneficial for tendon/ligament injury and can be useful in combination with my manual treatment. An example is that in many cases I find it quite important to help the patient improve the efficiency of their movement patterns (including occupational usage) to avoid further injury.

In addition, there are many other methods besides these three by which tendons and ligaments are treated in both standard and complementary medicine. While many have some positive effect they are often limited in treating the serious, chronic injuries that are the focus of this book. These conditions generally do not reach a positive outcome with most therapies. This book will discuss the standard medical treatment because it is received by the most patients in this society. That discussion provides a clear reference point for viewing my approach.

The central topic of this book is presented in part as a research study determining the effectiveness of my therapy model for chronic injury. Case studies from my clinical work will be used as a primary example, and related to scientific findings and theories. This helps to provide an overall vision of the book's variety of material.

## Sequence of the Book

Main features of the book are linked here to its progression.

The nature of tendons and ligaments is featured in Chapter 2. This reveals important insights into physiological healing processes of these structures. Portrayal of their composition and function is basic for looking into injury and recovery. Here is a foundation for the case studies and the entire topic. Primary information about these connective tissue structures begins Chapter 2, and will lead to the conventional medical perspective on their function and healing capacity. We next see recent scientific research findings and theory that alter and expand the widely accepted outlook.

In the standard model ligaments and tendons are relatively passive. Recent information and outlook demonstrates a more active, vital function. There is a general sense of the dynamism of body tissues. Creative concepts of tendons/ligaments are originated by such researcher/clinicians as Bainbridge Cohen, Korr, F. Smith, R. Becker, Hunt, and Studitskii. Their theories amplify scientific research findings on the health aspects of connective tissue neural involvement, electromagnetic activity, cellular function, and its process of tissue regeneration. Ideas for effective manual therapy methods, exercise, and other health-enhancing strategies clearly emerge from this material.

Chapter 3, "A Manual Therapy Model for Tendon and Ligament Injury," describes my therapeutic approach. This includes a view of the various techniques and the skills and aptitudes needed to apply them effectively. The chapter opens with an outline of the standard medical treatment for tendon and ligament injury that is so widely utilized in this society. Its prevalence makes it an important reference point for viewing my working strategy.

There is an overview of each of the principal techniques in the model and an explanation of how I use it to address an injured tendon or ligament. Select essential principles are common to all the techniques. Another section compares my approach for these injuries to that of the standard model. In dramatizing the central points and overall scheme of the two strategies the comparison gives a reader a perspective on both, and on non-surgical conservative care in general. This can be a practical clarification of important factors for success with difficult injury cases.

The techniques section presents main features and fine points of the techniques, and usages that are both regular and unorthodox. It has many instructional elements and can be useful to clinicians in a number of ways, although it is not a total training manual. It will be informative as to how and why a method is employed and where it is particularly beneficial (especially for tendon/ligament injury). Although this does not preclude what I regard as the necessity of learning one or more of the techniques very thoroughly, it does illustrate how techniques in combination can be utilized effectively for injury cases. Portrayal of the individual elements (techniques, knowledge) and their interweaving into an overall approach that makes up this model may afford readers from various backgrounds a sense that can also be applied to a range of structural (and other) health issues.

A vital element of my working strategy is the abilities and aptitudes that are used to apply the manual techniques. My route to learning these skills and methods is chronicled in a discussion of personal background and professional training. The account provides some illustration of how and why the model has been developed in this form. One major influence is my own recovery from a serious tendon injury.

The first two case studies in Chapter 4 are thorough accounts of the course of therapy for a serious, chronic tendon injury and a corresponding ligament injury. These are information-rich cases selected for an in-depth look. They are examples of essential aspects of tendons and ligaments and my usage of the manual methods. After each account, there is a case-progression chart tracing a sequence of variables over the course of therapy. Fifteen additional case accounts form the chapter's last section, adding breadth and showing a variety of situations for using this approach. Cases involve injuries from sports, workplace, accidents, and overuse.

The main variables traced in the cases are 1) comfort/pain, 2) range of motion, 3) level of function, and 4) clinical findings such as tissue quality of the tendon/ligament. These are central to in the book's research study which evaluates therapeutic efficacy of my approach, with conclusions drawn in Chapter 7. The beginning of the fourth chapter introduces the research, providing a perspective on the case accounts which are the main part of the chapter.

Chapter 5 views the processes and tissue changes as a tendon or ligament recovers from chronic injury. It is timely to see a systematic look at how their structure and function changes in healing. This receives little coverage in most available writing. The reader sees how each of these changes can be promoted by methods from the therapy model—showing a more fully textured sense of the recovery process related to a conservative care (non-surgical) method.

Chapter 6 offers self-help strategies for ligament or tendon injuries. While this is not a substitute for professional treatment of serious injuries, it can be a useful adjunct. The chapter has guidelines for a four-stage, step-by-step strategy of exercise and rehabilitation from onset of injury to recovery. The second half is advice on sports injuries, prevention, and recovery.

Chapter 7 is an overview and a discussion of the case studies. It relates these accounts to primary topics such as healing capacity of tendons/ligaments and vital changes for recovery. The cases are seen in light of various aspects of my therapy model. There is a section of further thoughts on important tools and abilities for a practitioner to effect positive results with serious injuries.

Chapter 7 presents conclusions and an overview related to the possibilities raised in the book for:

• a more potent healing response of ligaments and tendons,

• a fresh view of health care principles in a new approach to chronic sports and overuse injury,

• benefits of manual therapy and its potential in serious cases.

My central focus in the book is a grounding in information on the above topics, leading to a sense of greater possibility.

# CHAPTER 2

# THE NATURE OF TENDONS
# AND LIGAMENTS

A range of information in this chapter provides insight for the entire topic. Material here on tendons/ligaments is vital for understanding injury, recovery, and the therapy I am using. The story of the dancer, Julia L., in Chapter 1 refers to my work with adhesions and laxity of her injured tendon and the alignment pattern of its fibers—and a steady recovery process. These physical changes are given a foundation in this chapter.

The material here reveals much promise for the potential of these connective tissues to heal. The account starts with basic structure and function. Following are standard medical views and then the perspective of innovative theory and research. This introductory preview and a chapter summary will acquaint less technically-oriented readers with the essentials of the material.

Grounding in the basic structure begins with a view of collagen fibers, cells (fibroblasts), and ground substance—building blocks of tendons and ligaments. This proceeds to their essential properties such as visco-elasticity and tensile strength. The passive structures seen in the conventional model do not produce movement; when stretched past a certain point the tissue cannot regain its normal resting length and will remain lax. When the process of injury becomes serious it results in major tearing of fibers, adhesions, tissue degeneration, and loss of function. Portrayal of the central, primary elements of inflammation and chronic injury syndrome can inform us as to how they can be reversed.

Following is a section featuring findings from recent scientific research enriching the standard perspective. Intriguing clues in this material lead to avenues through which manual therapy can benefit the injured structures. Normal connective tissue (e.g., tendons and ligaments) continuously remodels itself for regular healthy maintenance. There is increasing evidence that these tissues are equipped to repair themselves from injury by manufacturing new microfibers and large amounts of collagen and ground substance.

Through new information the traditionally held view of the neural function of ligaments is expanded to a more active one; they are involved in complex neuromuscular feedback circuits. Data indicates that the richly innervated, responsive tendons/ligaments play a substantial role in neural control of movement and posture. Research in electromagnetism points to its important bodily influence on internal reporting of and response to injury, along with growth for repair. Connective tissue appears to react readily to this form of energy, which is also linked to the acupuncture system. This has intriguing implications for its healing potential and for treatment strategies, as does research on the properties of cells.

Studies in cell biology yield evidence for contractile capacity of non-muscle cells, including the fibroblasts of tendon and ligament tissue. Cellular contraction and capacity for locomotion indicates strong possibilities of the tissue to generate forces from within itself. Such activity could increase tissue tone when it is weak and also assist reversal of laxity; this lengthened condition of chronically overstretched ligaments is usually thought to be irreversible without invasive procedures.

Other potentially valuable cellular aspects of connective tissue health are found in research on satellite (stem) cells. These relatively simple cells are active in regeneration of damaged muscle. A cellular cycle of despecialization into stem cells, leading to their respecialization in order to form healthy tissue, may be operative for injury reversal in all body tissues. The conditions that promote regeneration are described as the "plastic state." This state is a component of a basic bodily healing response, seen in the chapter summary.

This chapter is a backdrop for the cases of the people reported in Chapter 4, and defines the whole topic. The latter part of the material here includes the insightful theories of some pioneering researcher/clinicians in the field. Their views on tendons/ligaments round out the chapter's picture of relatively dynamic, interactive structures. From my standpoint, there is some fascination with the scientific evidence of vitality and sophistication embodied in these tissues.

## Structure, Composition

Tendons and ligaments are dense, regular connective tissue structures (bands, cords, or straps) with mostly parallel fiber arrangement. Connective tissue has much variety, but in general it is characterized by the presence of a large extracellular matrix and a wide dispersion of cells.[1,2] The *cellular* portion of tendons and ligaments are the fibroblasts that synthesize and maintain the fibers and the ground substance.

The *extracellular* matrix consists of ground substance and fibers. The ground substance is the nonfibrous component of the matrix and is made up of glycosaminoglycans and proteoglycans. These long-chain molecules are linked to the collagen fibers to help form connective tissue. The ground substance facilitates tissue metabolism and provides support, shock absorption, and resiliency. It also decreases friction and attracts and binds water. Water occupies the largest percentage of weight (and space) in all tissues (60% to 80%).[3] The varying percentage of water-binding protein contained in the ground substance affects the hydration level of the tissue.

The fibrous component of the matrix is primarily collagen fibers, with some elastin. This is the support framework and comprises 75% to 80% of the dry weight of tendons and ligaments. Collagen is the most abundant protein in the human body; its basic building blocks are amino acids, primarily proline, glycine, and lysine. Its amino acid chains assemble into long triple helix molecules by hydrogen bonding to oxygen radicals along the chains.

The collagen molecules line up side-by-side to attach by intermolecular bonding, forming the hollow collagen fibers. These fibers are the individual units that also attach by molecular bonding to form fascicles (bundles) that comprise the overall structure of the tendon or ligament.[4,5] Cross-linkages between molecules and fibrils are electro-chemical bonds important for structural strength of the tissue.

Collagen fibers have a tensile strength approaching that of steel. The parallel arrangement of the fibers is somewhat wavy in the relaxed state, and straight when under a tension pull. Dense connective tissue has more collagen fibers and less ground substance than other connective tissue. Elastin is an extensible substance that forms a small component of tendons and most ligaments. A low percentage of specialized ligaments contains a large component of elastin, which gives them increased extensibility.

Tendons and ligaments are surrounded by a sheath (called a paratenon, and unnamed for ligaments) of loose areolar connective tissue, which facilitates gliding on contiguous structures. In locations involving high-friction forces, particularly in the wrist and hand,

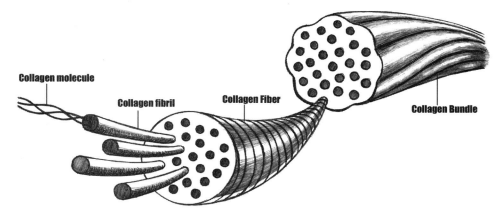

**FIGURE 2**
Collagen structures in tendon or ligament.

tendons are surrounded by an additional sheath beneath the more fibrous paratenon. This is the epitenon and is a synovial tissue layer that produces synovial fluid for lubrication.[1, 6]

Tendon tissue blends with muscle at one end, and at the other (similar to both ends of a ligament) meets with its bony attachment by blending through the fibrocartilage covering, and then into the cortical bone itself.[7] The musculotendinous junction and tendon-bone, ligament-bone junctions are often the location of injury. Ligaments are extra-capsular, intra-capsular, or are thickenings of the joint capsule. Both structures are richly innervated and have relatively little direct blood supply.

**FIGURES 3A AND 3B**

Ligaments and tendons in location. The iliolumbar ligaments (3A) contribute to stability of the lumbosacral area. Therapy for a biceps femoris tendon (3B) injury (Julia L.) was described in Chapter 1.

## Properties, Function

The following description of the properties and function of tendons/ligaments represents the accepted view in standard medical theory. Some aspects of this view are altered in the perspective of recent theory and research. Ligaments are described as passive structures whose main function is to stabilize joints, guide their movement, and prevent excessive joint motion.[7] Tendons are also described in the standard literature as passive structures. Their main function is to transmit forces from muscle to bone and fascia.

Collagen structures are described as anisotropic, as they don't have equal mechanical properties when loaded in different directions. They exhibit properties (strength and elasticity) that vary according to their orientation in space when a constant force is applied.[1, 8] Due to their parallel fiber arrangement, tendons and ligaments are particularly adapted to resist tensile loads.

Ligaments and tendons exhibit the property of visco-elasticity. Similar to purely elastic materials, they can regain their original shape following deformation, after removal of the deforming load. When an elastic material is stretched it has work done on it, which increases its energy. It stores this energy and keeps it available, which enables the material to recoil back to its original shape. Due to the additional presence of viscosity, visco-elastic materials exhibit time-dependent properties of recoverability. Connective tissues also are temperature sensitive, which affects their rate of creep (slow elongation). To most effectively stretch out (elongate) this tissue, it should be heated and subjected to a large load over a long time period, to produce creep.[1, 6, 7]

When tendons or ligaments are subjected to sudden, prolonged, or excessive forces, the elastic limits of the tissue may be exceeded and the tissue enters the plastic range. In the plastic range the tissue is permanently deformed and is no longer able to return to its original state following removal of the deforming force. Ligaments or tendons that are thought to be incapable of returning to their original length after elongation are described as lax, or permanently elongated.[1, 7] After the plastic range is exceeded, with continued loading, the structure reaches the point of failure as the fibers rupture.

The term "load" refers to an external force applied to a structure. Two main factors determine the strength response of a ligament or tendon under loading: their size and shape, and the speed of loading. The greater the number of fibers that are oriented in the direction of loading, and the wider and thicker those fibers are, the stronger the ligament or tendon. These structures exhibit increased strength and stiffness (resistance to movement) with an increased speed of loading.[1, 7, 8]

Tendons and most ligaments have a fairly balanced combination of brittleness (resistance to force without having a plastic range) and ductility (capacity for deformation without failure). They have some brittleness and some ductility. Differing values for failure point are given in many references, but Frankel's and Adams' figures are fairly standard when they state that collagen fiber bundles reach a failure point after exceeding an elongation of either 6% to 8%[7] or 10% to 15%.[9] This is typical for tissue with a very high percentage of parallel collagen fibers (tendons and most ligaments). Tendons and ligaments have a high degree of resilience—the capacity to absorb and store energy within the elastic range, and then readily return to the original dimension and release that energy.[5] Their normal response to intermittent tension (application and release of a tensile force) that is not excessive is an increase in thickness and strength.[1]

Connective tissue ground substance can vary from a watery sol-state to a viscous gel-state. It has the characteristic of becoming more fluid when it is stirred up, and more of a solid gel when it is colder and sits without being disturbed. With a higher metabolic rate, motion, and warmth, the energy level of the tissue is raised and the ground substance is more fluid and ductile. With a lower energy level from reduced metabolism, lower temperature, and inactivity, the ground substance is more of a gel and the tissue is less able to soften and stretch.[5]

When tendons and ligaments are subjected to prolonged immobilization, they show disorganization of their parallel fiber arrangement and a decrease in their water and proteoglycan content.[3, 7, 10] The tendon or ligament insertion into the bone becomes weakened due to osteoclastic activity destroying their fibers. In some tests, ligaments that had been immobilized for eight weeks showed decreases in strength and measurements of load-to-failure of 35% to 40%.[3, 10, 11]

## Standard Medical View
## of Properties, Capacity for Healing

The standard medical model of the properties and healing capacity of ligaments and tendons is that which is most prevalent for orthopedists, sports medicine physicians, and some physical therapists. In this perspective these structures are seen as passive structures that don't inherently produce movement. Their tension is dependent on their length. Ligaments are described as "fixed-length stays."[5, 6, 7, 12]

Viscoelastic properties are recognized, and when stretched so that their deformation is increased to the point of failure they will not be able to return to their original dimension (length). There is little or no discussion of any other property that would reverse this laxity. Paris states that overstretched ligaments cannot regain tone, making it difficult to correct poor posture.[13] Subotnick's view is that fibrocytes (mature fibroblasts) of adult tendons are inactive, so that healing is dependent on metaplasia of surrounding fat cells.[14] The standard view is that once an injury is chronic, laxity cannot be counteracted by conservative care and can only be reversed surgically.

A characteristic opinion is expressed by the surgeon who states that "once a ligament is torn it is never going to come back all the way" (even with surgery).[15] Ligamentous fiber rupture is seen as difficult to heal, and is usually treated by surgery. Likewise for a tendon, the greater the extent to which it is torn, the higher the probability that surgery will be recommended.[6, 7, 8, 13, 14, 15] The medical perspective is that if tendinitis becomes chronic, the tendon gives way to scar and degenerative tissue and can require surgery to clean out the area.

Substantial rupture of the Achilles tendon will most often need surgical repair. Seeking to downplay unrealistic expectations of the possible results of surgery, Garrick states that "there are injuries that just don't get better" (even with surgery).[15] There are variations as to when an injury is defined as chronic. The orthopedist Keene defines a chronic tendon injury as one with over six to eight weeks' duration.[8] Definitions of chronic injury extend to being over six months' duration, with three or four months as fairly common.

The standard medical view of tendons and ligaments and their injuries determines their treatment in most instances. The clients in my case studies had exhausted the standard care options and had then chosen not to undergo surgery.

## Neural Involvement: Standard View and Recent Research Findings

The traditional view of the innervation and resultant function of tendons and ligaments has been altered by information from some research findings since the 1960s. Ligaments are intimately related structurally with the joint capsules and have similar neural receptors. In most of the cutaneous sense organs and joint areas, the receptors are specialized, histologically modified ends of sensory nerve fibers.[2] They convert energy into action potentials. The four cutaneous senses are touch-pressure, cold, warmth, and pain. Traditionally, the receptors identified by anatomists in joint areas are the Ruffini, Pacinian, Meissner's, Merkel's, and more recently, free nerve endings. All these are mechanoreceptors that respond to tactile stimuli. The tendons contain receptors known as Golgi tendon organs, which have close correlates found in ligaments.[2]

The traditional view was that ligaments had some of the same receptors contained in joints, and that these articular receptors function to provide some proprioception (sense of body position in space) and a protective role of supplying signals in a reflex loop with neighboring muscles. When the ligament or joint reaches the end-point of movement range it reports through paths to the spine, which in turn effect muscle contraction through stimulating the alpha motorneurons in the muscle—thereby providing a splinting action preventing further joint movement.

Recent research findings lead to a new perspective. Ligaments and joint receptors are now also seen as part of a more complex neuromuscular control system, which also operates through the smaller gamma motorneurons, located in neuromuscular spindles (stretch receptors) embedded in muscles. When the gamma neurons receive appropriate signals related to position and movement range and rate, they effect contraction of the muscle that they supply.

The gamma loop is a length-regulating reflex mechanism for each muscle that is protective against excessive stretch; it is important for production of accurate, well-coordinated movement and postural control. Its functions have been brought to light relatively recently. Ligament and joint receptor signals have considerable effects on this feedback system.[16, 17, 18, 19] They affect it throughout the entire range of joint motion, and include rate of movement as another reporting variable in addition to position.[16, 19, 20]

Swedish neurophysiologists Johanssen and Sjolander report on research findings showing that joint and (particularly) ligament receptors are able to report joint angle throughout the full range of movement.[20] The presence of mid-range receptors expands on the older model that restricted signaling to the end-points of range, and shows that articular receptors contribute more substantially to movement and position sense than was previously recognized. It has also been shown recently that the complexity and diversity of articular receptors are equal to that of cutaneous receptors.[17] In addition there is now strong evidence of rich

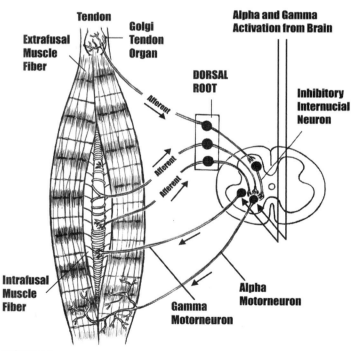

**FIGURE 4**
Muscle spindle and gamma neuromuscular loop. This illustrates the schema of the gamma nerve fibers supplying the intrafusal fibers of the muscle spindle, alpha nerve fibers to the main (extrafusal) body of the muscle, and their connections with the central nervous system. The drawing indicates the influence of muscle spindle activity on the main muscle fibers.

innervation of ligaments with the same nerve types as those in joint capsules, to provide varied receptor flows through the whole range of joint movement.

Nerves are now seen to fulfill an important trophic function of providing delivery of nutrients to peripheral structures such as tendons and ligaments. Korr and other investigators have elaborated this mechanism.

Neurotrophic activity, the delivery of proteins by axoplasmic flow from the nerve cell body along the axon to its target tissue (both antegrade and retrograde), varies in the rate of flow and quality of the axoplasm.[16, 39] It can be compromised by structural pressures in the nerve root, along the course of the axon, and in the target tissue; it has major effects on the health of tendons and ligaments, which are so richly innervated.[16, 54] Freedom from excessive structural pressures is necessary for optimal trophic function.

These recent research findings indicate an expanded neural role for ligaments and tendons. Ligament and tendon receptors function to assist smooth coordination of movement and muscular contraction for stability, as well as contributing to position and equilibrium maintenance through signaling to the brainstem and supplying higher centers with input related to more conscious body-image.[21] Much of the nerve control of posture is located in tendons and ligaments.[17, 19] In many ways they are highly sensitive structures that play a more important neural role than is portrayed in the traditional view. This role is more responsive and complex.

## Injury Process and Result, Tissue Changes

Depiction here of injury and inflammation primarily has conventional acceptance although some of the information is recent (Korr, Simkin, Radin, Viidik). It is a foundation for expansion and alteration of the standard view that resumes in the section on tissue remodeling, through the end of the chapter.

There are some common features and characteristics of the process and result of most tendon and ligament injuries. Injuries are most likely to result from a sudden trauma, or to be more gradual and then be classified as some type of overuse injury. There are also systemically caused injuries from disease such as rheumatoid arthritis or diabetes, endocrine imbalances, or from infection.[7] A tendon injury is termed tendinitis, a ligament injury usually called a sprain. Inflammation occurs, causing abnormal and impaired function of the tendon or ligament. There is some degree of rupture to the fibers and blood vessels of the structure, and some swelling. Tendinitis can often involve damage to the tendon sheath.

Establishing a diagnosis includes examination for instability of the joint where the tendon or ligament is located, and examination for loss of function.[8] Radiographic findings can be utilized. Injuries are often classified into three grades reflecting degree of rupture and instability.[6, 7, 8] In Grade 1 injury the ligament recovers its resting length after trauma and sustains microfailure of some fibers. In Grade 2 the structure doesn't completely recover its length, and there is some instability and a greater degree of fiber rupture. In the Grade 3 injury the tendon or ligament has a region of gross disruption of its fibers, and considerable instability. The serious injury thus consists of significant fiber tearing and loss of function.

Traumatic injury to a tendon often occurs when there is sudden unanticipated stretching of an already contracted muscle, resulting in a tear of its tendon. Likewise, an unanticipated force applied to a ligament incapacitates its afferent signaling to limit joint motion via muscle antagonist contraction. Thus, the joint may undergo a substantial, sudden movement and the adjacent ligament can rupture.[22]

Gradual onset (overuse) tendinitis is caused when microfailure of fibers occurs from excessive repetitive loads on a tendon, or when the rest period between loads is inadequate to enable the tendon fibers to regain their resting length. Predisposing influences are temperature extremes, excessive vibration, repetitive tasks, tissue degeneration, or usage in unusual postures.[6] Chronic injury processes and the degenerative tendon changes pictured in the "What My Hands Told Me" section of this chapter are important in overuse/repetitive strain problems.

Tendinitis (or ligament sprain) often starts as minute single-fiber tears. When the fibers tear they also swell. This causes them to rub against the tendon sheath, which becomes irritated and can also swell. The capacity for tendon gliding in the sheath is reduced as more and more adhesions are formed. Progression of the problem will result in a greater degree of tearing. It is common to find nodules, fatty mucoid deposits, and marked thickening in the ligament, along with a chronic low-grade inflammatory process[4] (see Figure 5, "Main Elements of Tendon/ligament Injury").

## Inflammation in the Injury Process

Inflammation is an important aspect of tendon or ligament injury. It is a term used for a large group of normal processes provoked by damage or alien material.[2, 23] Inflammation is in part a bodily response to injurious agents in order to remove toxic or foreign material. Fiber and blood vessel rupture in injury leads to infiltration of the region with white blood cells, platelets, fibrin, histamines, blood, and tissue fluids.[24, 25, 26]

Inflammation manifests as swelling, heat, redness, and pain. The acute inflammatory phase lasts from three to seven days after injury. Following this acute phase the result is either tissue repair or adhesion and scarring (see upcoming section on remodeling process).

When the inflammatory process is prolonged, it causes problems for the ligament or tendon that is healing.[26] Continued inflammation leads to excessive adhesion, fibrosis, and scarring. There will be inappropriate cross-linking of the fibers which contributes to dense, inflexible tissue. The developing fiber orientation is often random and scattered (not parallel).[23]

When lymphatic drainage is inadequate, the continued edema from excess fluid results in decreased circulation from excess pressure.

Edema in the joint area disrupts alignment and contact of the bone surfaces that leads to joint instability and consequent increase of ligamentous laxity. The rheumatologist Simkin reports that continued joint inflammation can compromise the capacity for lymphatic drainage, which further compounds the problem of instability.[24, 27] False strain reflexes caused by long-term inflammation result from excessive afferent nerve input to the CNS. The excessive input is partially caused by musculoskeletal tension imbalances, and also acts to maintain them (see section on neural involvement).[28]

When a region remains swollen the structures are bathed in serofibrinous exudate. Fibrin, a protein needed in blood clotting, is deposited between tissue layers in tendons and ligaments, and between them and surrounding structures such as sheaths. The fibrin seals these structures in a shorter, less mobile, adhered condition.[2, 29]

The purpose of post-injury vascular events as part of the inflammatory process is to mobilize and transport the defense components of the blood (leukocytes) to the injury area, and to secure their passage through the vessel walls into the tissue spaces. When this post-injury defense mode is prolonged excessively, it interferes with the normal healing process of the tissue. A self-perpetuating cycle of irritation and inflammatory response leading to further irritation becomes a component of the chronic injury pattern.

## Chronic Injury

In chronic tendon and ligament injury, the normal healing process of connective tissue is disrupted. Normal tissue remodeling is prevented by stresses (such as prolonged inflammation, inactivity) and hypovascularity.[8, 10, 25, 26] Connective tissue tends to become shorter and denser as it heals, unless it has beneficial conditions.[30] This contracture and thickening partially results from the increased interfiber bonding in a shortened state. The individual fibers lose gliding capacity and mobility relative to each other as do bundles of fibers, and whole tendons and ligaments relative to their surrounding structures (joints, capsules, sheaths).

Normal condition

Laxity

Tearing

Adhesions

Misalignment

Degeneration

**FIGURE 5**

Main elements of tendon/ligament injury, disruption of fibers. A combination of two or more of these patterns would be found in a chronic injury.

The adhesion process of fibers and layers of tissue leads to reduced extensibility and mobility.[1, 5] With poor circulation, hypoxia, and continued tearing, tissue regrowth takes the form of scar tissue as tears coalesce in portions of the ligament.[10, 26] Scar tissue is weaker than the normal type. The water content and amount of ground substance (proteoglycan content) of the tissue is reduced; there is a lessening of its normal ratio of ground substance to collagen fibers, which is another factor causing a denser, less pliant structural situation and impaired metabolism of the tissue. By-products of tissue degeneration and breakdown can form deposits in the ligament, disrupting its function.

In chronic injury the normal parallel fiber arrangement is disorganized, which reduces extensibility and strength. Prolonged low-grade inflammation is maintained along with disturbed lymphatic and vascular flow. This also causes abnormal metabolic function in the tissue.[8, 26] Ligaments and tendons can exhibit both hypo- and hypermobility. Often, both these conditions exist in different portions of the same structure. There is a disruption of balanced neural activity, as the tendon and ligament receptors report inappropriate strain signals caused by the irritation of the tissue.[16, 31] This sets up an ongoing stress on the ligament due to muscular tension, uncoordinated movement, and joint instability; all these factors contribute to general neurotrophic disturbance and impairment of circulation in the tissues.[16, 20, 31] An in-depth look at degeneration change in an injury process is seen ahead in the "What My Hands …" section.

## Remodeling Process of Connective Tissue

In normal nonpathologic functioning, all connective tissue is capable of healthy remodeling. Rolf asserts that it is in a continuous state of structural reorganization.[30] This self-renovation is exemplified by the response of tendons or ligaments to increased stress levels. Tissues respond to fatigue stresses (such as athletic training) by increasing the rate of tissue production (collagen fibers, ground substance). When there is proper vascular function and tissue metabolism, and sufficient rest between loading, the body can adapt adequately.[1, 7, 25, 32]

It is important for healthy remodeling of a ligament or tendon that the fibers are laid down in proper alignment. Non-excessive, well-directed loads on the structure with adequate rest encourage the healthy alignment of the fibers. The result is a structure that is stronger and also properly deformable, with adequate inter-fiber mobility. Good extensibility is also facilitated by remodeling with a normal ratio of collagen to ground substance. (It is important to have enough ground substance in the proportion.)[6, 23, 25] Production of ground substance is readily stimulated by movement after a ligament has been immobilized.[82]

The acute inflammatory phase immediately following an injury (described earlier) is the first of a three-phase post-injury healing process. Acute inflammation lasts from three to seven days and is followed by a proliferative/repair phase.

The proliferative (second) phase includes ingrowth of capillary buds and the appearance of fibroblasts that start to manufacture ground substance and collagen. The combination of new blood vessels, fibroblasts, and extracellular matrix is termed granulation tissue. The proliferation phase lasts until about the 21st day after injury (although it can be longer as the three post-injury phases overlap each other).

The third phase of the post-injury process is maturation/remodeling. It usually starts at 14 to 21 days and can extend a year or more. Collagen production continues and now is greater than that of ground substance. Remodeling includes the chemical cross-linking of the fibers which enables them to gain fuller strength. Type 3 collagen formed in the proliferation phase is replaced by Type 1 collagen which forms stronger fibers.[23, 26, 103, 105]

There is now increasing evidence that connective tissues are equipped to repair themselves by manufacturing and remodeling large amounts of collagen and proteoglycans. These components are continuously, although slowly, remodeled in the tissue in its normal healthy condition. When an injury occurs, production of connective tissue (along with collagen and proteoglycans) can double or triple. Synthesis of collagen by the fibroblasts is given a high priority (for nutrient supply in the body) during the healing process. Fibroblasts are responsive to extra-cellular influences such as cytokines, growth factors, and inflammatory mediators that allow fibroblasts to maintain and repair connective tissues. Fibroblasts are capable of proliferation to repopulate a region.[99]

## Blood Supply of Tendons

In their book, *Tendinitis: Its Etiology and Treatment,* Stanish et al. synthesize research findings on the blood supply of tendons, which had previously been thought to be avascular.[102] The tendon receives blood supply from three avenues, each serving about one third of the tendon:

1. Musculotendinous junction. Small blood vessels divide near the junction and send branches to both muscle and tendon. There is no

direct capillary circulation between muscle and tendon except that some vessels in the outer covering of the muscle (perimysium) traverse the junction.

2. Along the length of the tendon. The supply is either from the paratenon or the synovial sheath of the tendon. The paratenon contains many vessels.

3. Tendon–bone junction. Tendon and bone vessels do not communicate directly. There are indirect anastamoses between tendon vessels and those in the periosteum.

Internal vasculature. Vessels are primarily longitudinal in the endotenon and thus arranged around fiber bundles (fascicles). Vessels are the size of arterioles and are flanked by two veins. Capillaries connect them. The internal vessels are fed by vessels in the epitenon which enter radially.

Vasculature of the tendon or ligament is reduced in areas of friction, compression, and excessive wear. Shearing and other forces can damage the vasculature. Reduced, compromised vascular supply is a major element in tendon injury.

## What My Hands Told Me: Clinical Experience and Current Research on Injury and Recovery

My perceptions in 29 years of palpation and observation are in line with the direction of much new investigation in the field. The case study reports in Chapter 4 illustrate my direct sense of damaged and healing ligaments and tendons as intricate, responsive, lively structures. In revising for this second edition, it is exciting to see that many research insights from the last four years further confirm and elaborate a more vital, complex picture of ligament and tendon metabolism, injury, and recovery.

Highlights of current research results in this section of the chapter are as follows:

• Further evidence that tendons and ligaments are more metabolically active than the traditional view. Research focuses on collagen physiology and production, the cross-linking process of collagen fibers, and the vascular supply of tendons reported in a preceding section. (Much of the newer research here targets tendons.)

• A shift of emphasis regarding tendon dysfunction and injury. The ongoing focus on the inflammation process in tendon injury has been expanded to a shared emphasis with the role of internal degeneration of the tendon. Research now provides a more detailed picture of the changes involved in degeneration and injury.

• As evidence of recent recognition of a somewhat greater healing capacity for tendons (and the need to counteract degeneration), a program featuring exercise has received attention in injury rehabilitation. There has been more investigation into the structural integrity of tendons and tissue changes in the strengthening process.

## METABOLIC ACTIVITY OF TENDONS

A recent increased awareness of tendon metabolic process is reflected by the researchers Stanish, Curwin, and Mandel which acknowledges this metabolic activity. They report that only recently has research interest been focused in this area because of long-standing beliefs that metabolic activity was negligible.[102] Several areas of tendon physiology are now more illumined.

## CROSS-LINKING IN COLLAGEN STRUCTURE OF TENDONS, LIGAMENTS

Curwin writes that the vital role of healthy cross-linking for proper strength of the tendon has now been given more importance.[103] These bonds are essential for adequate tensile strength in the tendon or ligament.[104] Cross-links can be damaged by shearing forces which occur in injuries. The process of link formation and maintenance necessitates adequate enzyme supply to the tissues, as well as sufficient oxygen supply provided by good vascular activity.

The cross-links are enzyme-facilitated chemical rearrangements of adjacent amino acids. They start as bimolecular, and in mature structures progress to trimolecular, a process that can take months to complete. The influences of both exercise and different types of collagen on cross-linking activity are discussed below.

## COLLAGEN PRODUCTION, PHYSIOLOGY

The continued metabolic activity over time of tendon/ligament cells, fibrocytes (tenocytes) is confirmed by Jozsa and Kannus.[105] Previously thought to be inactive, fibrocytes are the successor to the more active fibroblasts, although the reverse conversion sometimes occurs. Some major features of recent research on collagen physiology are:

• Curwin's study of the effects of exercise (jogging) shows that tendon collagen cross-linking increases with gradually increasing loads, but actually decreases with intermittent strenuous loads. She reports studies concluding that collagen tissues can be induced to form new microfibrils which can group together to form new fibrils. The new microfibrils can also be added to existing fibrils, increasing their size.[103] There is now added validation that exercise increases collagen synthesis, concentration of metabolic enzymes, and the size, number, and strength of fibers.[102, 103, 106, 107]

• Collagen has several types, of which the primary component in normal tendons is type 1 collagen. Type 3 collagen is found abundantly in degenerated tendons and those healing after injury, and is normally less than 5% of a healthy tendon. Type 3 forms smaller diameter fibrils, and during healing converts to type 1, which promotes more cross-linking, forming larger, stronger fibers.[103, 105, 108, 109]

• Increased load-bearing capacity in tendons results from collagen bundles sometimes following a more complex three-dimensional structure which is not solely in the straight longitudinal alignment. Studies now show spiral and diagonally-oriented bundles in portions of some tendons, which is well suited to their demands for force transmission.[105]

• Cellular response to mechanical forces on connective tissue is the subject of some new studies. Injured rat tendons treated with mechanical pressure from solid instruments exhibited fibroblast proliferation. The cells in these tendons also showed signs of fibroblast activation and active collagen synthesis such as increased presence of rough endoplasmic reticulum, larger numbers of ribosomes, and prominent round nuclei.[110] Mechanical stretching of fibroblasts also stimulates their proliferation.[111] While ultrasound treatment produced regenerative response of connective tissue in some studies, others such as Almekinders' showed no sign of regenerative effect.[105, 112]

• Ruptured fibril ends in tendons can be rejoined by synthesis of new collagen materials.[105]

## INJURY PROCESS—RECENT PERSPECTIVES

The role of degeneration is now featured more prominently as a major factor in tendon injury. The earlier parts of this chapter emphasize an inflammatory process in connective tissue dysfunction, and we currently have more insight into inflammation as it interacts with degeneration in ligaments and tendons.

Tendinosis has now joined tendinitis as a description of injury. Tendinosis refers to intratendinous degeneration that can initially be asymptomatic.[6] It is non-inflammatory although it can interact with and overlap inflammation, and views vary as to sequence. Tendinosis is a process of atrophy-related factors such as vascular compromise, hypoxia, aging, microtrauma, overuse, tissue breakdown, and lack of adequate cell response.[102, 103, 105, 108, 113]

The two major types of tendon and ligament problems are overuse injury and substantial rupture; degeneration is now thought to be a frequent causative factor for each one. In overuse injury it is common that tissue microtrauma and breakdown (tendinosis) precedes the perception of pain. Pain usually signifies an inflammatory condition (now called tendinitis by some authors). Jozsa and Kannus studied tendons which had spontaneously ruptured within the preceding 24 hours. They found that 97% of the specimens exhibited significant degenerative changes.[105]

As pictured earlier in this chapter chronic dysfunction often involves a circle of inflammation, scarring, hypoxia, and failed healing response. The current view expands on earlier findings and includes a sharper focus on the elements of tendon degeneration and chronic disturbance. These elements are:

• Vascular compromise leads to hypovascularity and tissue hypoxia. The result is impaired metabolic activity and tissue nutrition.

Studies show compression from stasis of extracellular fluid and narrowing of the lumina of the arterioles. Deposits of fibrin and thrombus formation are found. Damage to the microvasculature can occur in localized regions of the tendon. Vascular compromise and insufficient oxygenation (tissue hypoxia) receive the highest emphasis as a central factor in tendon degeneration.[105, 107, 114]

• Fatty deposits can be intracellular, in tenocytes, disrupting cellular oxidation. Lipid deposition also occurs between fibers leading to disrupted alignment and fiber separation and thinning. Unhealthy accumulations of mucoid ground substance deposits lead to similar problematic effects as from the lipid deposits. Portions of the tendon can exhibit a soft, mushy consistency.[105, 113]

**Figure 5A**
Degeneration, failed healing tissue. This is a composite showing:

1. "bubbles" at center and upper right
2. mucoid vacuole at lower left
3. fibrin granular material
4. lipid droplets (ovals)
5. disruption and fraying
6. angulation. Loss of continuity without systematic orientation
7. bulbous amianthoid fibers
8. variations in thickness
9. loose structures

• An incomplete, failed healing response leads to accumulation of excessive fibrin deposits. These deposits can contribute to major disorganization of the internal structure of the tendon. The immature fibrinoid tissue in the tendon as well as buildup of degraded collagen, ground substance, and vascular granulation tissue is sometimes referred to as "amorphous debris."[102, 115]

- Collagen fiber alterations in the injury process include findings of bulbous fibers as well as thinned, frayed, split, curled fibers. Fibers lose continuity as there are microruptures of tendinous bundles. Strained or ruptured tendon fibers exhibit tapered ends and knot formation, both consisting of denatured collagen. Hypoxic changes in the tendon lead to progressive increase in the dryness content of its collagen fibers, increasing fiber stiffness.[105] Fibrosis, adhesions, nodules, and scarring are common in tendinosis and have been covered earlier in the chapter.

- Cross-linking of fibers is impaired by inadequate oxygenation, enzyme defects, and endocrine response to stress (which may result from athletic overtraining).[103] Progressive collapse of lateral cohesion from inadequate cross-linking results in more loss of strength and vulnerability in the tendon.

- Cellular abnormalities in a degenerative process include lessened numbers. Decreased cell response capability results from tissue overload and hypovascularity. This diminished capacity of the cells to respond normally is a primary cause of degeneration. The cells (fibrocytes) exhibit altered nuclei and nucleoli, dilated vacuoles, swollen mitochondria, reduced DNA, and dilated degranulated endoplasmic reticulum.[105]

- Calcium deposits (hydroxyapatite crystals) appear in the tendon, partly as a result of hypoxia in the tendinosis process. There is also a non-degenerative, very painful, rapid onset condition of the shoulder, termed calcific tendinitis.[116] Wolf describes his success in calcific tendinitis with a technique of needling into the calcium deposits to treat this acute condition.[117]

- Inflammation and its central role in tendon or ligament injury is illustrated in detail earlier in this chapter. Inflammation can cause degeneration and rupture and can also result from overuse and degenerative changes. Recent studies suggest that inflammation can be initiated by the presence of calcium deposits, fibrin deposits, and degraded, denatured collagen in the tendon and its sheath.[115] The inflammatory reaction may be an auto-immune response.[118] Stanish et al. feel that pain indicates ongoing inflammation of a tendon/ligament and is the most common measure of tendinitis severity.[102]

## OVERUSE INJURY

Overuse is now thought to account for 30% to 50% of sports injuries.[104] A high percentage of occupational-related patients also present with a slow, insidious onset consistent with much overuse tendon injury.[108] All the degenerative tendon changes listed in this section can occur in overuse conditions. Overuse tendon and ligament injury (repetitive strain injury) can be defined as a level of repetitive microtrauma sufficient to overwhelm the tissue's ability to adapt.[119]

## EXERCISE PROGRAMS FOR TENDON REHABILITATION

Exercise programs to promote tendon injury recovery are now receiving more research interest and validation. This emphasis is consistent with the view that degeneration and its reversal is important in tendon injury. Exercise can be beneficial for promoting collagen synthesis, remodeling, and tensile strength.

Eccentric exercise, where tissue tension is generated as the muscle-tendon unit lengthens (e.g., lowering a weight) is a vital component of some recent programs. Eccentric (lengthening) contraction produces a greater force in the muscle and tendon than concentric contraction. A number of authors feel that many sports injuries occur in the eccentric phase of the activity cycle. Eccentric contraction is more efficient than concentric in that the muscle uses less energy and recovers more quickly.[120, 121, 122] A 2001 study for treating Achilles tendinosis showed superior short-term results for eccentric calf muscle training compared to concentric training.[123]

A program featuring eccentric exercise for tendon injuries has been created by Stanish, Curwin, and Mandel at the Sports Clinic of Nova Scotia.[102] This program (described more fully in Chapter 6) has reported good clinical results as has a related program used in Swedish and Danish controlled-trial research studies.[106, 124] The subjects in both the Swedish and Canadian studies had utilized physical therapy and conventional exercise programs without success. Curwin's article offers perspectives on the appropriate application of their program; her view is that all joint signs should be cleared and the subject should have a pain-free range of motion before starting the program.[103]

Both Peter Edgelow, P.T., Clinical Professor of Physical Therapy at UCSF and Diana Herold, Dance Medicine Director at St. Francis Hospital Center for Sports Medicine, feel that the eccentric exercise program can be helpful for patients at a certain stage of recovery. It could be a useful component of an overall program.[125, 126] Edgelow, an expert in treating thoracic outlet syndrome, emphasizes for rehabilitation the need to restore coordination and balance as much as strength. He feels that the eccentric phase of movement enhances control and coordination more than the concentric phase.

For areas with more complex biomechanics such as the shoulder, more guidance is beneficial for the patient to do eccentric exercise along the best line of direction. There is a need for more limited range of motion exercise in earlier and/or more severe phases of injury, that can include some eccentric training.[126] An eccentric exercise program for tendinopathy is presented in Chapter 6.

## LIGAMENT INJURY REHABILITATION—RECENT DEVELOPMENTS

Much of the material in this section on research developments is primarily focused on tendons, although it is very likely that a high proportion of findings on collagen physiology and injury/degeneration also applies to ligaments. While we are still waiting for more attention to ligaments in the literature, some recent information includes:

• Reports of success for ankle sprain exercise therapy using an "unloading technique" (harness suspension, incline board) to reduce gravitational force and allow pain-free exercise.[127]

• Balance, proprioception, and strength training reduced risk of re-injury after ankle sprain.[128]

• Friden et al. found impaired proprioception in the knee joint after ligament injury.[129]

- An engineering model study shows the anterior cruciate ligament can be injured differently at varying knee joint angles.[130]

- Loosli and Oshimo's study demonstrates that a thorough exercise and bracing program had equal or greater success compared to reconstructive surgery for effective rehabilitation of anterior cruciate ligament injury in recreational athletes (tennis, skiing).[131] Dancers' knee injuries responded well to specialized Pilates exercise.[132]

## HEALING POTENTIAL—RECENT PERSPECTIVES

A healing capacity of tendons and ligaments that is greater than the traditional view now has further confirmation from researchers. Stanish and Curwin discuss the current reassessment of a long-held attitude that connective tissue healing is "slow and imperfect." Their exercise program is based on acceptance of significant tissue remodeling capacity of tendons.[102]

Jozsa and Kannus feel that recent evidence shows that tendon healing capacity may have previously been underestimated. They describe how denatured collagen and frayed fibril ends in tendons are readily removed by proteolytic enzymes produced by macrophages. The ruptured fibril ends may then be rejoined by the synthesis of new collagen materials.[105] A Scandinavian study reports the regeneration of Achilles tendons after necrosis.[133]

The material on collagen physiology in the preceding pages includes aspects important to the recovery process. Among them are: the capacity for tendons to develop new microfibrils which form new fibrils or thicken existing ones, fibroblast activation and proliferation in response to mechanical pressure, continued long-term activity of tendon/ligament cells (fibrocytes), and validation that exercise can increase collagen cross linking and synthesis. Exercise increases production of insulin-like growth factor (IGF-1) in tendon fibroblasts. IGF-1 is known to strongly stimulate collagen synthesis and cell replication and seems to mark remodeling activity.[114]

A presentation on stem (satellite) cell activity in connective tissue appeared in this book's first edition, and is a subject which is now receiving a tremendous amount of interest for regeneration of many types of tissue. Discussion of stem/cell activity is found in the upcoming section on tendon and ligament regeneration.

## Electricity, Magnetism, and Tendons/Ligaments

A number of researchers in the last three decades have found evidence demonstrating the presence and influence of electricity and magnetism in connective tissue function. This appears to have an effect on the health status of tendons and ligaments and their capacity for healing from injury.

**Ependyma lines cavities of brain and spinal cord**

**Nerve**

**Nerve fibers**

**Schwann cells surround all nerve fibers**

**Nerve fiber or axon**

**Figure 6**
Direct Current conduction system in perineural structures.

Orthopedic surgeon and researcher Robert Becker describes a bodily Direct Current system of internal communication, located in the perineural cells that ensheath the entire nervous system including the brain.[33, 34, 35] Becker traced the DC internal field map as it mirrors the design of the nervous system. This was confirmed by studies using the SQUID device for magnetic field detection.[33, 36, 37] It is an analog communication system that integrates body processes and controls the activity of the body's cells by producing DC electrical environments. The analog DC system is more primitive than the digital AC system of nerve impulse conduction, and can provide a relatively steady-state environment interacting with AC activity. Becker and others found this system to have an important role in growth and healing.[38, 39, 137]

The Direct Current circuit flows appear to guide formation of collagen after tissue injury.[34] Dr. Becker describes a "current of injury" that is a DC flow from injured tissue that serves as a reporting mechanism. This conveys information of bodily damage to the brain and can evoke a response that is vital to reparative growth and other internal controls (see Figure 8). Magnetic energy was found to be increased at the location of injury.[33] The Swedish radiologist and researcher Nordenstrom also reports evidence demonstrating an electrical current circulatory system in the body switched on by infection and injury.[40] The cell biologist Lackie's research indicates that a wide variety of individual cells appear to have the ability to respond to DC fields.[41]

Williamson reports on tracing magnetic fields from the body that are produced by activity of potassium ions along cell membranes. He also asserts that ferromagnetic substances in the body can interact quite strongly with the geomagnetic field.[37] Becker reports on research showing the influence of the geomagnetic field on bodily growth patterns, stress responses, and biological cycles.[33, 34]

The physiologist and researcher Valerie Hunt describes a "growing emphasis from biomagnetic field studies on the electrical nature of life."[42] Motoyama and Reichmanis have both researched and demonstrated specialized electrical characteristics of the acupuncture meridian system.[40] Reichmanis found it to be linked to the perineural DC system and showed that acupoints generate DC potentials.[43] Hunt's research found acupuncture-like meridian energy flows in all connective tissue. She describes connective tissue as an anatomical electromagnetic circulatory system. The microtubular array of collagen in connective tissue is a structural component that facilitates this conduction.

Hunt's instrumentation detected differing electromagnetic currents in various body tissues. Denser tissue like bone and cartilage exhibited slower moving, lower frequencies that she associates more with direct current and magnetism. (This in comparison to "lighter" tissues like nerves and glands with higher frequencies and more alternating currents.) Tendons and ligaments as denser tissue exhibit the predominance of the magnetic part of the field.

Dr. Hunt characterizes the magnetic part of the spectrum as that which is instrumental in tissue healing.[42] She found that the energy at the location of an injury switches from predominantly electrical to become primarily magnetic in preparation for repair and healing. The increase of the low frequency magnetic field encourages repair cells to redifferentiate and grow. She notes the similarity of the repair role of this direct current flow to that which is described by Robert Becker. Hunt asserts that a primary breakdown in the body's healing response can occur in the electromagnetic system—in the strength and range of its impulses, as well as in its coherency. This appears to have a major influence on the condition and healing capacity of connective tissue including ligaments and tendons.

## Contractile Capacity, Cellular Locomotion

Information that expands the conventional model until this point has been in the areas of neural involvement, bioelectromagnetism, and self-remodeling of the tissues. Another broadening of the perspective on the properties and functional capacity of connective tissue is provided by examining research on its contractile capacity and its cellular motility.

There is evidence for the widespread existence of the structural components and the active mechanism for contractile capacity in non-muscle cells. Cell biologists and biochemists have found a system of muscle-like proteins in nonmuscle cells, including fibroblasts. These proteins are actin, myosin, tropomyosin, and actinin. Actin is one of the body's most abundant proteins, constituting between 5% to 15% of the total protein content of cells.[2, 41, 44, 45] Actin can self-assemble into a helical polymer filament. Myosin is a hexamer and not a single protein.

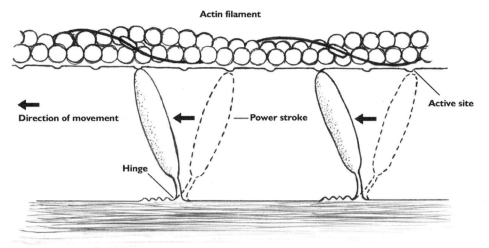

**FIGURE 7**

Actin-myosin motor.

The interaction between actin and myosin is basic to what is termed the *acto-myosin motor,* which is a primary contractile mechanism vital for muscle contraction. A primary component of this process is myosin filaments containing protruding heads, which are potential cross-bridges. The myosin heads fold/unfold as they attach and release by molecular bonding with various sites on the actin filament. This causes a pull that moves the actin. This contractile motor mechanism is found allso in nonmuscle cells, including fibroblasts.[41, 45, 46, 47]

*Cell locomotion* occurs when the cell moves its position relative to its surroundings, and is the most sophisticated of cellular movements. Studies on tissue fibroblasts and large amoebae have provided much of the evidence for the mechanism of crawling movement of cells.[41, 44] The process includes a phase in which actin assembles into a cross-linked gel meshwork in the "front" or protrusive portion of the cell. This protruding region of the cell adheres to an anchorage beyond the present distal sites, so that the contractile machinery can pull the cell forward.

Cell locomotion thus involves two main components: 1) the acto-myosin motor system to generate contractile forces, and 2) an actin gel-assembly process for protrusion of the front of the cell. The cell surface must have the capacity for attachment, de-linking, and then reattachment to a new site. Locomotion of fibroblasts is essential for wound healing. The fibroblasts move into the area and then the contraction of numbers of fibroblasts pulls the edges of the wound together.[41, 44]

Evidence for the mechanism of cellular contractile capacity and locomotor activity of nonmuscle cells, when applied to the fibroblasts of ligaments and tendons, indicates that these structures may not be as passive as was previously thought. Tendon and ligament tissue would possess the capacity to generate motion from within. This changes the perception of them as inert, passive structures that are only moved by external forces.

The evidence would also indicate that the tissue has some capacity to reorganize itself into a different shape and to contract in ways that would facilitate the knitting together and condensing of tendons and ligaments that have been overstretched; these would have previously been considered to be permanently lax.

## Possibilities for Tissue Regeneration in Tendons/Ligaments

To discover capabilities for tissue regeneration of injured tendons and ligaments, I have explored research findings for regeneration of various body structures; this provides a view into basic mechanisms of the process. There appear to be common features that are applicable to tendon and ligament healing. Extensive research in this area was done by Robert Becker in connection with his investigation of bioelectricity, but first is a look at the regeneration and repair of muscle tissue by satellite cells.

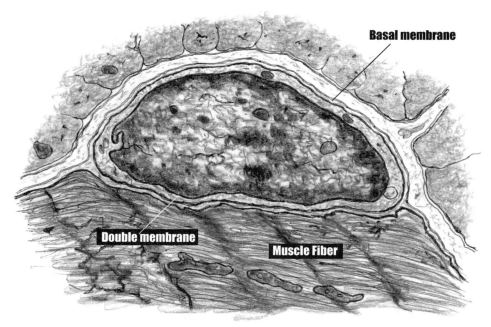

**Figure 8**

Satellite cell located in periphery of muscle fiber.

The satellite cell in skeletal muscles was discovered by Mauro in 1950 and is the *stem cell* (unspecialized), which, when activated, provides a new cell population for muscle regeneration in vertebrates by transforming into myoblasts.[48] They are small mononuclear cells below the basement membrane, stored in the extra-cellular matrix of the muscle fiber.[49, 50] The Russian histology researcher Studitskii reports that "transformation of satellite cells into myoblasts is now an established fact."[50] This is particularly distinct following trauma, and may be instrumental in normal development and self-renovation of muscle fibers.[49, 51]

The two theories of satellite cell origin are: they are myonuclei that are pinched off from damaged muscle cells which then de-differentiate to form a population of myogenic cells, or they are an ongoing reserve of precursor cells below the basement membrane.[52] They have the ability to synthesize DNA, divide, generate differentiating muscle cells, and give rise to new stem cells.[53] Under steady-state conditions stem cells are quiescent.[53]

The result of satellite cell activation is development of daughter muscle fibers in maternal ones, and subsequent separation into new fibers. The molecular biologist and muscle researcher Richard Strohman reports that satellite cells can form new fibers or activate the thickening of existing fibers. This occurs not only after major damage, but in conditions of increased loading of the muscle where a normal repair function leads to strengthened fibers.[48, 49] He feels that normal growth and regeneration are different degrees of response along the same continuum.

Studitskii did extensive studies on skeletal muscle transplantation and grafting and the role of satellite cells. He defines plasticity as the capability for structural change depending on change of conditions. This is a different usage of the word from the description of "plastic range" of tissue deformability described earlier in this chapter. The plastic activity of muscle tissues is manifested by structural changes of growth and differentiation; it is facilitated by a particular reactive state of the tissue that Studitskii calls the plastic state.[50] The *plastic state* appears with any condition that deprives the muscle of its working capability, including weak traumatization. Plastic activity is a restorative phase that in muscles involves the appearance of satellite cells.[50]

My sense is that the concept of the plastic state and the conditions that favor it provide a very useful insight into successful strategies for connective tissue healing. There are some factors that *favor plastic activity* of muscle. These include hypervascularity (including ingrowth of blood vessels) and hyperinnervation of the tissue and surrounding areas. Activation of conditioned reflexes brought about by massage or exercise of the contralateral or adjacent muscles stimulates the plastic state.[50] Studitskii used various methods of interrupting the working activity of the muscle (including some irritants) to produce the state. Strohman finds that introducing a highly erratic stimulus activates stem cell growth.[49]

Passive stretch appears to be another facilitative influence on plasticity.[51] Both a high basal metabolic rate and adequate local tissue metabolism are helpful to plastic activity. Strohman reports his findings that local (hormone-like) growth factors in the tissue can activate satellite cell activity.[48] Studitskii emphasizes the importance of nerve influence (including trophic activity) for maintaining optimal metabolism of an organ or tissue and for facilitating the plastic state.[50]

Dr. Robert Becker's research findings on the perineural Direct Current system of control and communication in the body were described earlier. Here is a view of his findings on regenerative growth, mostly with electromagnetism in regeneration of limbs in vertebrates, and bone fracture healing in humans.[33, 34] He defines regeneration as the formation of complex body parts involving growth from simpler into more complex cells (redifferentiation). Physiological repair is defined as cell proliferation of the same type, which heals wounds by closing the gap. This is distinct from a wound being patched over with scar tissue.

Becker identifies two basic stages of regeneration. The first stage starts with wound clean-up, which culminates in the de-differentiation of nearby cells to form a blastema. A blastema is a mass of primitive embryonic cells appearing at the site of an injury. De-differentiation is the process in which a mature, specialized cell returns to its original, embryonic, unspecialized state, and

**DC system control center in the brain**

**Input signal**

**Injury**

**Fibroblasts make collagen fibers**

**Sensitive cells de-differentiate**

**Figure 9**
Direct current injury response and growth control system.

apparently is stimulated by magnetic and DC flows after injury ("current of injury"). In the second phase, also stimulated by DC flows, the embryonic cells pile up as the blastema elongates; they then redifferentiate and take their proper place.[34]

Invertebrates can regenerate entire limbs. Becker theorizes that mammals cannot because they seem to lack two elements necessary for the first stage of regeneration (see above). One is that there is a shortage of cells sensitive enough to de-differentiate in order to form a blastema. The second element is that mammals lack a high enough ratio of nerve to limb tissue to produce adequate strength of the electrical stimulus needed for de-differentiation. However, he devised some successful strategies for facilitating the phases of regeneration in mammals by applied electromagnetism. This was particularly notable in facilitation of fracture healing in humans.

Becker's research does show that collagen, so abundant in tendons and ligaments, is a piezo-electric generator, and also that collagen fibers can align in parallel in response to a weak DC flow. He feels that the potential repertoire of human cells is greater than is now realized and that there are possibilities for tissue regeneration that have not yet been actualized.[33, 34]

There are some important similarities in the findings concerning the essential features of tissue regeneration, when Becker's work is compared to that of the researchers on muscle regeneration involving satellite cells. Both approaches describe a process wherein there is cellular de-differentiation into unspecialized cells (or in some cases the appearance of unspecialized stem cells from other sources), which subsequently redifferentiate into specialized cells for tissue production and maintenance.

The muscle regeneration and electromagnetic research have each found that it is vital to have adequate nerve currents in the tissue. Both have also found that regeneration is favored by a healthy, strong metabolic function in the tissue, facilitated by adequate vascular and lymphatic flows. Although tendon/ligament regeneration is not their main focus, Studitskii does mention findings that the localized fascias and tendons have a high degree of plasticity during muscle regeneration and that they repeatedly reorganize until a final structure is formed.[50]

A direct focus on connective tissue healing (and its involvement with cellular differentiation from simpler cells) is found in the work of the Danish cell biologist A. Viidik. His research indicates that connective tissue wound healing involves fibroblasts that are derived from undifferentiated perivascular mesenchymal cells, some of which come from the small blood vessels supplying the tendon or ligament.[26] Certain conditions that encourage the plastic state are available for tendons and ligaments, and would seem to favor their healing process. Viidik states that regeneration of the original tissues in connective tissue injury is not exceptional, and cautions not to assume that healing by scar tissue formation is the only possibility.[26]

Aside from the issue of cellular transformation, the fibroblasts themselves are active cells that can produce large amounts of collagen and ground substance. They are very active in wound healing and are capable of proliferation to repopulate a region.[99] Studitskii finds that fibroblasts play a major and essential role in the regeneration process.

An interesting perspective on the capabilities for tendon and ligament repair and regeneration is presented by the movement analyst, educator, and occupational therapist Bonnie Bainbridge Cohen. The educational/therapeutic approach she has developed, Body-Mind Centering, includes a segment of working with tendon and ligament problems; this reflects her view of these structures as being more responsive and functionally active than in the conventional model. Body-Mind Centering is empirically derived from 1) observation of sensing movement patterns and of clinical data, and 2) comparison of this with standard anatomical knowledge.[55] Regarding regeneration, Bainbridge Cohen believes that it is possible to reach a source of de-differentiated cells and activate them to effect de-differentiation.[56] She describes a structural matrix of the ligament that is comprised of small latticelike, electromagnetic hooklike connections. These "hook-ups" can realign into their innate pattern in response to therapeutic input, and effect significant tissue reorganization and healing.

She feels that overstretched, damaged tendons and ligaments can regain most or all of their proper tone, length, and thickness.[55] Their fibers can regain their proper spacing (proximity) and alignment. They can knit together, or loosen as needed. She states that conventional approaches have little idea of the actual possibilities for dramatic change of structure.[56]

Bonnie Bainbridge Cohen sees the role of ligaments as providing guidance, efficiency, and clarity to movement and alignment, and setting a pattern for muscular response.[55, 57] The ligaments provide an automatic movement control, and (as Basmajian also says) they fatigue more slowly than muscles, thus playing a vital role in weight-bearing and maintenance of posture.[21] Her view is that one can initiate movement from the tendons or ligaments, and that activating the ligaments adds to movement clarity and range. The activation will decrease muscular effort and tension. It is important to use the ligaments in movement. Body-Mind Centering uses a manual therapy approach that is extremely specific and detailed in its treatment of tendons and ligaments. She feels that there is some contractile capacity of their tissue and that they have a contractile function.[56, 57] Bainbridge Cohen's perspective is that the traditional view sees ligaments as too passive; they have a fuller, more active role and healing capacity.

## Summary

Structure, properties, and function of tendons and ligaments are described in this chapter. We have seen the process of tendon/ligament injury and the anatomical and physiological changes in continuing dysfunction. The normal remodeling process of healthy connective tissue portrayed in this chapter is a foundation for the recovery process. Many of these elements are at work in the situation of the dancer's tendon injury in Chapter 1 and in the cases of people to be reported later.

The standard medical view of ligaments is that they are passive rubber band-like structures. They are seen as "fixed-length stays" whose neural function consists of some proprioception and involvement in a simple reflex loop system that provides protection for the joint.

Research findings demonstrate that ligaments (and tendons) are more active structures having a significant role in weight-bearing and postural control, ongoing active cellular function, responsive to electrical and magnetic activity, and containing tissue components possessing some contractile capacity. These findings show a relatively extensive neural role for these structures with involvement in the gamma motor system and substantial provision of vital afferent input to the CNS. This is essential to coordination of movement and posture. Some functional aspects of ligaments seen in these research findings are favorable factors in potential for healing from injury.

The standard medical view of the injury healing capacity is that once it has been stretched beyond the limits of the plastic range, a ligament becomes permanently lax and cannot regain its normal tone and structure. A chronic injury consisting of a significant degree of fibrous rupture of a tendon or ligament is considered to have little or no possibility of recovery without surgical treatment. Surgery itself often does not have a favorable prognosis for promoting full, lasting recovery.

Increased healing capacity for tendons/ligaments is indicated in recent research. We can be encouraged by the chapter's evidence for the factors listed below.

Factors that enhance tendon/ligament repair described in this chapter appear to comprise a *basic bodily healing response* that may function in any area. These elements are reactions to injury, promoting the healing process. While many factors also lead to recovery, the following list emerges from the research findings and theory in the preceding pages. A basic healing response for an injured structure is:

• Appearance and/or proliferation of the types of cells in the injured tissue that are necessary for its repair. I have mentioned stem cell (less specialized) activation that leads to re-differentiation into specialized cells. Another possibility is proliferation of characteristic cells (e.g., fibroblasts) in the tissue.

• Acceleration and intensification of normal tissue renovation and remodeling to restore a healthy structure (reversal of tissue degeneration and the proliferation of fibroblasts in response to injury mentioned above are examples of this mechanism in connective tissue).

• Activity of hormone-like growth factors in the inflammation stage and repair process.

• Electromagnetic activity involving an electrical current circulatory system (this may be a perineural Direct Current control system) responding with a "current of injury." This can guide tissue remodeling and encourage the reparative function of the cells.

• Neural feedback circuits connect to the central nervous system and promote healthy autonomic and somatic neural control of metabolic and movement/postural activity for the injured area.

• The "plastic state" promotes tissue regeneration. Plasticity here is the capacity for structural change. This particular reactive state of the tissue appears in response to injury and in muscle involves activation of satellite (stem) cells. Plastic activity is facilitated by several factors including plentiful vascular and neural activity in the injury area, along with high basal metabolism and adequate local tissue metabolism.

In addition to the elements of a general healing response, there are other specific factors that can promote tendon/ligament recovery. One factor is the contractile and locomotive capacity of some of their tissue components, along with connective tissue motility (generating of forces from within).

The continuous metabolic turnover and remodeling process (self-renovation) of connective tissue are also health-enhancing influences. Collagen tissue appears to have capacity for repairing its torn microfibers and producing new ones. Plentiful neurotrophic supply of nutrients to the injury area can promote recovery.

Certain therapeutic strategies emerge from the referenced sources that would encourage the mechanisms that allow tendon and ligament healing. These can enhance all the processes I have described as elements of healing response. For the chronically injured structure the strategies are:

a) Increase its oxygenation

b) Raise its metabolic rate (energy level of the tissue)

c) Ensure adequate vascular and lymphatic flow

d) Reduce inflammation

e) Remove excess waste material, deposits from the tissue

f) Promote healthy cross-linking of collagen fibers

g) Normalize the electromagnetic climate of the body region

h) Restore normal mechanics to the adjacent joints

i) Establish normal, balanced patterns of afferent input from the joint and tendon/ligament

j) Restore an adequate quantity of its ground substance (ratio of ground substance to fiber)

k) Reestablish the normal mobility and alignment of the individual fibers and their bundles.

Chapter 5 depicts these anatomical/physiological changes occurring as the structure heals, as they may be promoted by manual therapy.

Findings of the various scientific researchers in this chapter are a basis for its view of tendons/ligaments' favorable factors and capacities for recovery. This view points to greater possibility for their healing from chronic injury than in the conventional model. Expanded healing potential is in line with research data and clinical theory of researcher-clinicians such as Becker, Bainbridge Cohen, Hunt, Korr, Curwin, and Stanish. The upcoming material on manual therapy and case study accounts will show how this chapter's capacities, favorable factors, and strategies can be utilized in a manual therapy approach to promote recovery.

# CHAPTER 3

# A MANUAL THERAPY MODEL FOR TENDON AND LIGAMENT INJURIES

This chapter features: 1) the skills and aptitudes necessary for this approach; 2) the various manual therapy techniques that are used in the model, including some unorthodox usages of these techniques specific to injury treatment developed by the author; 3) essential principles of the techniques; 4) comparison of my treatment model with the conventional medical methods, especially standard physiotherapy; 5) my personal background as it relates to the model. Initially, as a reference point to a new approach, is the following outline of the conventional medical treatment received by the majority of patients in this society.

## Conventional Medical Treatment

Traumatic injury to a tendon or ligament is initially treated by rest, ice, compression, and elevation. Use of a splint or support will protect and rest the tendon and thus promote healing. Nonsteroidal anti-inflammatory drugs (NSAIDs) such as aspirin, Ibuprofen, and others are used to reduce swelling. After the acute phase or in longer-term gradual onset injury, contrast baths with alternating warm water and cold water are employed to improve local circulation. Devices are used that limit the motion range of the structure (e.g., a heel lift to treat an Achilles tendon injury).[8]

As pain and swelling subside a stretching program for the injured structure is started, using both passive and active range of motion. Other physiotherapy procedures used are whirlpool baths, ultrasound, and electrical stimulation.[58, 60, 61, 100] Strength training for the neighboring muscles includes isometric and various forms of isotonic resistance exercise. Massage techniques can be used, including transverse friction (cross-fiber) for the tendon or ligament.[25, 62] Various forms of manual joint mobilization are sometimes performed by the physiotherapist.

Cortisone injections for the injured tendon or ligament are sometimes utilized to reduce inflammation. There is some controversy around this procedure due to evidence that it causes atrophy of connective tissue and possible rupture of the tendon.[7, 14, 26, 63] Long-term use of NSAIDs may retard the healing process. Viidik states that use of anti-inflammatories, including corticosteroids, can be a cause of prolonged inflammation in connective tissue.[26]

Surgical techniques for musculoskeletal injuries can be categorized as either repair or removal. The orthopedic surgeon Garrick's view is that in general there is a higher success rate for removal operations, (e.g., removing bone spurs or fragments in a joint or thinning adhesions of an Achilles tendon sheath) In another surgical technique, holes are drilled in the nearby bone to stimulate circulation to the tendon. Most surgeries for tendon or ligament injuries are repairs.[7, 8, 136] In describing reconstruction surgeries for damaged anterior cruciate ligaments of the knee, Seedhom mentions: 1) primary repairs, 2) reconstruction with different tissues, 3) reconstruction with various synthetic devices.[11]

Frankel describes various forms of primary repair surgeries in which the tendon or ligament fibers are woven together. The end-weave method, which is strongest, has the disadvantage of being bulkier and possibly inhibiting gliding on adjacent structures.[7] In reconstruction using natural tissue, those used are: autogenous tissue (e.g., tissue from the patient's iliotibial band or patellar tendon for ACL repair), allografts using tissue grafted from a cadaver, or xenografts from bovine tissue.

Repairs with synthetic materials use polyethylene, polypropylene, and carbon fiber. The synthetic repair can be a complete replacement, a supplement to a natural tissue graft, or a scaffolding that encourages ingrowth of the patient's collagen tissue.[11] While many patients have been returned to their accustomed activities by these repairs and there is often at least a short-term relief of discomfort, Garrick states that after surgery, a tendon or ligament never recovers completely and that some don't recover at all.[15] A surgical procedure can be the best choice for some people and it is not focus of this book to advise on this question. Problems with the mobility and neuromuscular integration of the neighboring joint can be short-term or long-term consequences of the surgery.[1, 64] Recovery procedures from surgery consist of a period of immobilization followed by the treatment procedures previously described.

## Skills and Aptitudes

Illustrating the author's therapeutic approach starts here with important abilities that are involved. This section describes these skills and aptitudes, often referring to the statements of some prominent osteopaths and allied practitioners. They are abilities that in my experience make it possible to effectively practice the techniques that are presented in the next section.

It is very beneficial to be capable of detecting small bodily changes and picking up strains at "micrometric levels" of measurement.[65, 66] This involves the perception of bodily movements from the smallest and most simple, to the most complex.[67] One detects a difference between old and new strains.[66] There is the capacity to detect and become attuned to the rhythms of the patient's body (e.g., breathing, Cranial Rhythmic Impulse), some of which are quite subtle.[68, 69]

A thorough knowledge of anatomy and kinesiology is indispensable to me. The practitioner needs a familiarity with the normal motions of the body,[67] a clear image of the normal joint articulations and their mechanics, and a knowledge of the position and purpose of each structure. This familiarity, combined with an understanding of body structure and function, enables the effective and useful comparison of the normal body with the abnormal,[70] and the interpretation of material into sound physiological reasoning.[66]

It is important to be able to establish contact with the body while disturbing its function as little as possible.[71] Developing the capacity of using a very light, neutral touch is favorable for fine perception, allowing both information and therapeutic change to come through to my hands rather than pushing to discern something in the tissues or to force changes.[69] One allows the body to give its opinion,[66] as restrictions in the body may literally attract the hand to them—and take the practitioner to the center of dysfunctioning patterns.[72] Sutherland, who originated osteopathic cranial therapy, advises the therapist to develop familiarity with using the least force possible to accomplish the objective.[73] Skill enables accuracy, as Barral states; only very slight forces are needed for effecting structural change when one is precise.[72]

There is a skill in being able to synchronize one's attention. While I am working, the aim of internal physical focus is a state of attentive, balanced relaxation throughout my body, including all the senses. The osteopath Jealous calls this "defacilitation" of the practitioner's CNS, which involves relaxed breathing and muscular relaxation.[68] Centering and stillness within the practitioner's own body enables attunement to the patient's rhythm. Magoun calls this meditation-like state "a rapport in the tissues between practitioner and patient."[71]

Bainbridge Cohen speaks of the capacity to direct or focus one's sense organs. Sensing and perceiving are not just passively receiving input, but when done with attention and discriminatory awareness, become a "dynamic activeness of perceiving."[57] Rollin Becker advises developing a "listening finger-touch," which is more than a passive laying-on of hands—becoming an alert, observational type of awareness.[66] This capacity of "listening," an active receptivity, is a vital element of my work that is integrated into every aspect of diagnosis and treatment.

The practitioner develops the sensitivity of the sensory receptors (mentioned in Chapter 2) of his hand. The potential sensitivity of the human hand to pressure, motion, and heat is extremely high, and far greater than usually realized.[74, 82] Mechanoreceptors, proprioceptors and temperature sensors respond to these stimuli as well as to vibration.[68] Barral asserts that there is considerable evidence for palpation of infrared radiation (heat), and concurs with Hunt that receptors in the hand are sensitive to a wide variety of electromagnetic wavelengths.[42, 74] It is very useful for the therapist to be able to perceive and interact with various aspects of the electromagnetic field of the patient. The hand's receptors are located in skin, deep fascia, in and around joints (ligaments, tendons), and in muscle spindles.

The references quoted in this section from these leading teachers demonstrate much of the "lineage" of my model. This proceeds from the pioneering Sutherland and Lippincott, who incorporated A.T. Still's beginnings of osteopathy, up to the present-day teachers who are quoted. These include Smith, with a direction from Chinese medicine, and Bainbridge Cohen, whose work stems from earlier movement educators such as Bobath and Todd.

To conclude with the aptitudes: it is important that the clinician can sense and encourage motion and mobility within the tissues as initiated by these living structures[66]—realizing that manipulation is no substitute for the body's own power.[67] I have aimed to follow in the style of treatment based on the principle of osteopathy being the art of provoking self-correction on the part of the organism.

## Techniques I Use for Tendon/Ligament Treatment

The principal methods in my model are the osteopathic techniques of Strain/Counterstrain, Cranial therapy, and Visceral Manipulation, combined with techniques from Body-Mind Centering. Their active use is seen in the injury cases to be reported. There is also a significant role for acupressure, Zero Balancing, and osteopathic Fascial/ Myofascial Release techniques. The end of this section describes Joint Gliding technique which has been developed in this author's practice to articulate joint surfaces and promote healthy function of the joint complex.

This section will describe the basic mechanism and features of each technique and discuss how I use it to address various aspects of tendon/ligament injury. Chapter 5 also relates these therapies to the specific processes and tissue changes that occur in injury healing.

*Strain/Counterstrain,* one of the major osteopathic manual therapy techniques, was originated by Dr. Lawrence Jones starting in the early 1960s.[28, 64, 75] I have made extensive use of it since 1977. It is a gentle atraumatic technique that corrects joint dysfunction through the use of positional release. I move the patient's body slowly in non-painful directions, guided by local decrease in tissue tension and palpatory tenderness (in an indicator or "tender" point) under my monitoring hand, to find the optimal position of release. The patient is supported in this position of comfort for ninety seconds. It is usually an exaggeration of an abnormal alignment pattern, and involves the purposeful shortening of one or more tense muscles around the problematic joint.

**FIGURE 10**
One of the Counterstrain techniques for the carpal joints involves positioning the wrist primarily in flexion, while monitoring the decrease of localized tension and soreness in the indicator ("tender") point under the therapist's finger. The weight of the subject's hand and arm is thoroughly supported to relax in the position of release.

As I locate and maintain the exact release position, the tense hyper-sensitive tissue near the joint feels like it softens and loosens. There is a sense of activation and an even current (of electricity and acupuncture energy) moving under my monitoring hand. Often, I palpate an activation of localized vascular pulsation that after some seconds becomes more quiet and even.

The positioning effects the reduction and arrest of inappropriate (excessive) proprioceptor activity by markedly shortening muscles that contain habitually overactive muscle spindle (stretch) receptors. This quiets afferent discharge from the spindle (as well as other mechanoreceptors in tendon/ligament or fascia) and normalizes the alpha-gamma loop firing pattern; that enables the balancing of muscular and other soft tissue forces around the joint which is being treated.[16] The gamma loop is discussed in Chapter 2 (see Figure 4). The positioning influences the CNS to gradually turn down the "alarm signal" level of gamma efferent discharge to the affected muscle, allowing the muscle to regain its normal resting length. This repatterning of local and regional neural and soft tissue activity enables the joint to regain healthy alignment and motion. I have found the technique to be very advantageous in treating a wide variety of spinal and other joint-related dysfunctions.

The use of Counterstrain technique specifically benefits an injured tendon or ligament by reducing excessive muscular pulls on it—as well as reducing pulls from fascial tensions, structural misalignment, and pressure on Golgi tendon receptors. My experience is that because it is so gentle, the technique is very helpful for treating fragile, injured, or hyper-reactive areas. Reduced tissue stress in the area leads to reduction of inflammatory fluid and improvement of fluid dynamics and metabolic activity.

The positionings also promote recovery by improving mobility and usage patterns of the joint (near that ligament) through normalizing patterns of afferent input and balancing ligamentous pulls on all sides of the joint. The employment of Counterstrain corrections of (spinal) segmental dysfunction reduces or eliminates the output of neural misinformation; this neural output involves reflexes to the CNS and also involves irritated mechanoreceptors and nociceptors in a tendon or ligament which is in that segmental circuit. In treatment of a tendon/ligament injury I have used Counterstrain and related positionings that shorten the injured structure to more effectively perform specific tissue work with it while it is in the shortened position (see the following description of Body-Mind Centering techniques). This seems to reduce excessive localized proprioceptor activity in the tendon, which effects change in itself and enables greater efficacy of other techniques that I am using while the tendon is in that position.

The therapeutic model of *cranial osteopathy* is based on the existence of an active, mobile craniosacral system consisting of the cranial bones and membranes, the spine and its membranes, and the cerebrospinal fluid. Originated by Sutherland in the early years of this century, the model includes the twenty-two bones of the cranium having joints with a slight mobility—and a reciprocal tension membrane system consisting of the spinal membranes connecting with the intra-cranial membranes. The therapy is described in works by Sutherland,[73] Magoun,[71] Frymann,[76] Gehin,[77] and Upledger.[101] There is a characteristic dual-phased motion pattern of the craniosacral system (cranial rhythmic impulse, or CRI) that is normally six to twelve cycles/minute. My work with the rhythmic fluctuations of this system (and its wave-like movement that is reflected through the whole body) is both diagnostic and therapeutic.

Restrictions and imbalances of the cranial structure are treated with gentle manual techniques, often consisting of the indirect approach. Indirect technique consists of encouraging the structural components in a direction exaggerating the existing imbalance by following the mechanical pulls and forces of that body region to what feels to me like a point of rest; this allows rebalancing and improved condition of the localized structure. Indirect technique is also utilized in Counterstrain and to some extent in all other methods that I employ. Also similar to Counterstrain is the basic premise of inherent self-corrective forces in the body; the body is a self-correcting organism.

My therapeutic usage of cranial osteopathy for tendon and ligament injuries includes the harmonizing of a peripheral structure (such
as a ligament) with the CNS through connections to the spine and cranium. For an injured hand ligament this strategy involves my freeing
the motion of the CRI to that ligament through the upper limb—connecting from the dural membrane of the lower cervical spine (from
which the ligament derives innervation).

**Figure 11**
A technique for working with the dual-phased movement of the cranial rhythmic impulse (CRI)
through the hip to the ankle and foot. Using gentle pressures, the therapist balances and synchro-
nizes the CRI movements (arrows) of external and internal rotation of the hip, connecting to the
lower spine—with the CRI motion in the ankle and foot. This method is used to synchronize motion
through an injured Achilles tendon in a case study in Chapter 4.

Another example of benefit for an injury would be the freeing of a
cranial structure such as the occipito-mastoid suture, having a beneficial effect on membranous tension in the upper spine, which connects
to fascial tensions going through to the ligament in the hand. The
usage of fascial unwinding (described later here) is included in cranial
therapy. In a more general sense, alleviating excessive tensions in the
cranium and spine relieves pressures on important neural structures,
which may effect changes such as reduction of excessive sympathetic
nervous system activity. This reduction can lead to improved circulation to the body periphery where an injured tendon is located.[64]

Bonnie Bainbridge Cohen's theoretical and clinical model of the role and healing capacity of tendons and ligaments has been described in the second chapter. Her system of movement analysis and training, anatomy/kinesiology education, and manual therapy is called Body-Mind Centering, and has been developed since the early 1970s. The foundation of Body-Mind Centering (BMC) is the exploration and repatterning of the major body systems (skeletal, muscular, organ, endocrine, nervous, and fluid) as they initiate and support movement.[57]

Her experience as an occupational therapist leads to this method's focus on neurodevelopmental movement patterns. Optimal structural alignment is promoted in relation to the movement repatterning. In practicing this technique the therapist aims to utilize a level of sensing and activation of structures (including tendons and ligaments) down to their more minute components (e.g., fibers). This fine perception and control is utilized clinically in the BMC manual therapy approach to tendon and ligament injuries that is the most structurally specific and complete of any that I have encountered.[55, 56, 57, 78] I have made extensive use of it since 1974.

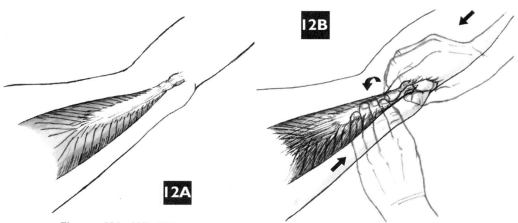

**Figures 12A, 12B, 12C**
Feeding in ends of a tendon alternated with drawing them apart. Therapy for a biceps femoris tendon injury was described in Chapter 1, and this techniques encourages proper alignment of its fibers. Figure 12A shows the tendon before treatment, with its adhesions and misalignment near the knee. Figures 12B and 12C illustrate the feeding-in phase of condensing the fibers longitudinally, which allows reorganization (see below). At the same time, the right hand is also used here with rotation to specifically aid realignment of a portion of the tendon which was particularly twisted (using indirect technique).

I use the BMC manual method of contacting both ends of a ligament (a similar method contacting the bony insertion and musculotendinous junction for a tendon), and alternately feeding these ends in towards each other and drawing them apart. For a shortened, thickened ligament the emphasis would be more in the drawing apart phase, and more on feeding in for a lax, weak ligament.

When a tendon is too short, separating the fibers perpendicular to their length will allow it to elongate. When it is weak and lax, unifying the fibers will allow it to condense. I alternate separating and condensing the fibers width-wise (perpendicularly) as well as longitudinally. This involves activation of what Bainbridge Cohen believes to be the perpendicular component of the microstructure of the tendon.

Bainbridge Cohen feels that tendon or ligament fibers naturally organize their structural interrelation with neighboring fibers by a "hooking" mechanism that creates a structural integrity. By manually condensing the ligament (longitudinally) one disorganizes the misaligned fibers and encourages this self-generated hooking activity. The

result is that the fibers are allowed to assume their natural organization. I find this similar to, and compatible with, the Counterstrain approach of placing the ligament in a shortened position. For a lax and weakened ligament the therapist positions the joint so the ligament is shortened, and concurrently uses direct manual contact with it to specifically encourage its fibers in knitting together and increasing its tone.

Additional clinical strategies of BMC that can be used for tendon/ligament injuries include a subtle manual contact through tissue layers to the capillaries in the area, in order to encourage healthy vascular flow in the tendon and its surroundings. This is done through gentle pumping action, which has the added effect of stimulating movement of the interstitial fluids in the localized zone.

**Figures 13A, 13B, 13C**
BMC techniques for increasing tone and substance, and decreasing laxity of the ulnar collateral ligament of the MP joint (seen in a later case study). The therapist is condensing the ligament from both ends as well as in a perpendicular direction. The schematic drawings (13C) show the ligament before treatment and as it is being condensed.

Repair is also enhanced by lessening strain patterns in bones adjacent to the injury area using BMC induction-type techniques; trauma or repetitive stresses can cause the various layers of bone to retain compaction and torquing that contribute to the unbalanced pulls on nearby structures. The clinician aims to activate direct movement initiation and create feedback and proprioception in the ligament. This activation of movement initiation in the injured structure is encouraged by the client's gentle movement of the adjacent joint, while I am focusing the movement in the ligament and offering a slight resistance. Resistance up to a certain level (and no more) will increase proprioception. The specificity and structural insight of Bainbridge Cohen's approach is of great value for my treatment of some fragile and stubborn connective tissue problems.

The osteopathic *Visceral Manipulation* techniques described and taught by Jean-Pierre Barral also aim at the normalization of reciprocal tensions throughout the body (as do all the techniques in the model). This includes some very effective assessment methods of "listening" for identifying the center(s) of these tensions. The treatments are focused on optimizing the structural condition and movement patterns of the organs of the pelvis, abdomen, and thorax.[67, 68, 79, 80, 81]

13C

Effective usage of Visceral Manipulation incorporates Barral's emphasis on anatomical precision. The techniques are direct and indirect low-force methods for freeing restrictions of the organs and their adjacent and surrounding connective tissues. These organs are structurally and functionally interrelated with the rest of the body through the fascial system and fluid and nerve pathways. It has often been my experience that a visceral restriction contributes significantly to a client's musculoskeletal problem (e.g., lumbosacral dysfunction) and that improvement of the visceral motion will result in definite benefit for the spinal problem.

Some examples of the method's use for tendon and ligament injuries are as follows: in addressing injuries in the upper limb I have often found it very helpful to use Barral's techniques for freeing the upper lobe of the lung, its pleura, and the strong connective tissue attachments of the pleura to the first rib, T1, and lower cervical spine[79, 81] (see Figures 14A and 14B). Injuries in the lower limb (e.g., Achilles tendon) seem to derive benefit if the clinician can free a lower abdominal/pelvic restriction such as limited mobility of the cecum or sigmoid colon. The general and local "listening" diagnostic methods in which the therapist allows his hand to be attracted and led to the important restriction are quite useful to me in clearly identifying regional structural dysfunctions in the tendon or ligament area.

Visceral Manipulation uses the technique of induction, in which the operator gently encourages the structural component(s) in the

**Figures 14A, 14B**
Technique for freeing restrictions of the upper lobe of the right lung, its pleura, and the connective tissue suspension of the top of the pleura. The clavicle is removed in Figure 14A to show the pleura's suspensory apparatus, which is being gathered by the therapist's left hand in Figure 14B. This induction technique is assisted here by the right hand's influence of slackening the tissue superiorly from below. The relaxed tissue may then exhibit pulls in various directions, which can be followed by the practitioner's hands.

direction of ease, least resistance, and greater motion, until a point of equilibrium is reached—and is then maintained until a release occurs in that structure (see Figure 14B). I have used induction (an indirect technique) to advantage in tendon treatment by following the pulls in the tendon fibers, and find this to aid in the correction of their alignment pattern. The technique responds to, and works to balance, the major force vectors in the tissues. It works to promote their balance and lessen their disrupting influence.

The acupuncture system of Chinese medicine includes a grid of energy pathways throughout the body called meridians or channels. The acupuncture points on these meridians have been found to be zones of lowered electrical resistance.[40, 43, 83] Acupressure therapy was the initial study in my career, and I now utilize it most often as a background to the structural work that I do. However, there are times that it is a primary focus, and some of these are for tendon/ligament injuries.

The meridian map is very useful for discerning and treating restrictions and blockages that are connected to the injured structures. Applying pressure on acupuncture points in the localized area (sometimes connected with pressure on distant points) facilitates the normalization and smooth flow of electrical and magnetic activity and current in the tendon.

Acupressure is also involved in the manual therapy system called *Zero Balancing,* originated by the osteopath Fritz Smith in the 1970s.[69, 82] He is also an acupuncturist, and has blended the two approaches to create a type of structural acupressure. The system is designed to free and enhance the movement of the ch'i (qi) energy through the body structure. This acupuncture energy flow has an electrical component, and I have found Zero Balancing useful in working with the electrical activity in tendons and ligaments. In Dr. Smith's model, the densest energy flow comes through the bones and the body's energy is most readily blocked at the joints.

The techniques apply sustained pressures ("fulcrums") and tractions (applied "vectors") designed to rebalance joints by interrupting their neurological feedback to the CNS and removing their blockages. Zero Balancing is focused on the clear identification of acupuncture energy movement, and enhancement of its flow through the joints (where tendons and ligaments are located). In my experience it is an effective systematic approach for combining beneficial structural change with normalization of acupuncture/electrical current. I have found that Smith's methods are useful as alternatives to, and in combination with, the Counterstrain joint positionings and can be very helpful for freeing joint restrictions in the locality of tendon/ligament injuries.

Many of the fascial planes of the body intersect at joints and I have found it essential to free the fascias in order to relieve excessive pulls and pressures on injured structures. All the techniques mentioned so far accomplish this to some extent, but I will now describe a specific method for addressing the fascias. I use osteopathic *Fascial Release* techniques, which also effect more optimal fluid and nerve function in the tendon or ligament by relieving strain on the fascial wrapping of vessels and nerves.[84, 85] The three major varieties of fascia (superficial, deep and subserous) form an interconnected reciprocal tension meshwork, which is the packing and wrapping of structures throughout the body.[5, 30, 85] The deep fascia can develop the most stubborn restrictions, as it is the densest layer. This deep layer forms the sheaths for tendons and ligaments.

**Figures 15A, 15B**
Fascial Release (indirect technique) can be used in combination with direct technique of stretching for the interosseus membrane, similarly for the flexor retinaculum of the wrist, which forms a boundary of the carpal tunnel. Figure 15A shows the retinaculum being condensed as one component of a Fascial Release technique.

Fascial Release Technique[84] is based on the principle of evaluating motion (of a joint or soft tissue) in all three planes and carrying it in the combined direction(s) of most freedom to a position of rest. The rest position is maintained until inherent movement restarts (or is subtly encouraged in the direction of ease), and the clinician follows in this direction with gentle manual pressure until there is balanced, free

**Figures 16A and 16B**
Figure 16A portrays a direct stretch of the interosseus membrane. Figure 16B is a schematic drawing of the interosseus membrane.

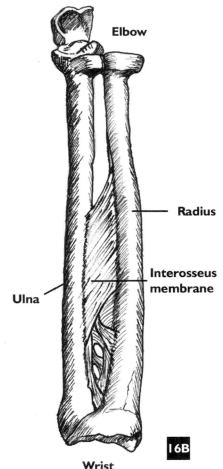

motion. This process is sometimes called fascial unwinding. In the course of freeing the restrictions of these tissues I find that there is sometimes also a release of memories and emotions associated with the physical pattern. This associated "tissue memory" is a common occurrence in the aftermath of high-impact injuries and its release can be helpful to the recovery process. I often combine Fascial Release (indirect) technique with direct techniques of stretching the fascial structures. The direct technique is very useful for zones of stubborn fascial binding and adhesion. It has been of vital importance for injury treatment to free the fascias, including the periosteum, in the close vicinity of the tendon/ligament. Recoil method (see page 167) is often included.

These techniques that I employ for treating the fascias are also very useful for *freeing restrictions in* the *muscles*. There is much structural interconnection: with perimysium wrapping bundles of muscle fibers, endomysium wrapping individual fibers, reticula entering the fiber, and septas separating groups of muscles. This configuration allows Fascial Release technique to be used efficaciously for muscle treatment, and it may appropriately be termed myofascial release.

The Golgi tendon organs near the musculotendinous junctions respond to changes in force (tension).[16, 86] Stimulation of these receptors effects an inhibiting neural influence on muscle contraction and causes the muscle to relax. I use the technique from Applied Kinesiology[86] in which the therapist applies direct pressure to the Golgi tendon organ to relax the attached muscle and return it to a more optimal resting length.

A crucial element of the recovery process is the relaxation of excessive muscle tensions that place abnormal strain on injured ligaments and tendons. This is accomplished by my use of the Fascial Release techniques, Golgi tendon organ pressures, and also by Counterstrain positionings. As described earlier in this chapter, the positioning shortens the muscle, relieving aberrant neuromuscular strain patterns, which allows it to then assume a more relaxed resting length.

Methods that I use for promoting normal, harmonious electromagnetic activity include manual pressure on certain acupressure points in the injury area and in areas adjacent to it. The smooth flow of electricity and magnetism is also facilitated by the cranial therapy approach of working with the CRI movement through the area of the tendon or ligament—sometimes connecting this all the way through to the spine and cranium.

I have developed a specific method of normalizing *electromagnetic activity* that consists of my feeling to discern if there is any sense of a blocked and overactive ("dammed-up") or a deficient electrical quality in the tendon. This can feel like the discontinuity and unevenness of "static" or uneven magnetic pulls. I then move the tendon tissue a small distance, to the placement that encourages smooth electrical current that flows through it freely in an increasingly steady, unpressured pattern. This placement also effects a sense of balanced, even magnetic pulls in the tendon. The positioning (which can be readjusted in the process of change) often involves condensing of the tendon or ligament fibers.

Electrical activity can also be balanced through applying manual contact on either side (proximally and distally) of a ligament or tendon. The therapist then applies a slight traction, compression, or rotational force between the two hands until the intervening flow of electrical current through the ligament is smooth, even, and balanced from one hand to the other. Another option is to apply mild direct, localized pressure to the ligament tissue until electrical (and/or magnetic) activity is balanced.

Some general findings are that weak, deficient activity often can be strengthened and increased by a light, shaking movement applied to the area, or stretching of the skin over the ligament. Tonification is also achieved by contact on either side (proximal and distal) that is used to apply a compression force by approximating my two hands (or fingers). Calming of "jangled," overactive electricity or magnetism in the ligament is promoted by applying mild traction through the area or applying gentle localized pressure to the tissue. These general guidelines may vary in different situations. When there is much compaction and tension in the tissue, one may need to begin by shortening it with contact from both ends (condensing) before traction can be applied.

**Figures 17A, 17B**
Electrical activity in a ligament. Figure 17A is of balanced, even current, and 17B of disrupted, non-coherent current. These illustrations are not numerical measurements. They represent a palpatory sense of this activity felt with my hands through manual contact with the ligament.

Iliotibial tract

Biceps femoris muscle

Biceps femoris tendon

Patella

**FOCUS OF TECHNIQUE**

Fibular collateral ligament

Head of fibula

Gastrocnemius muscle

Peroneus longus muscle

18A

**Figures 18A, 18B**
Working with weakened, damaged zone of left hamstring tendon. Left hand is gathering surrounding structures in direction of zone at tips of 2nd and 3rd fingers of right hand. Right hand anchors and supports distal portion of tendon, and is also in position for specific fiber work with the localized zone. Figure 18A shows a normal hamstring tendon (right leg), indicating the zone being addressed in Figure 18B.

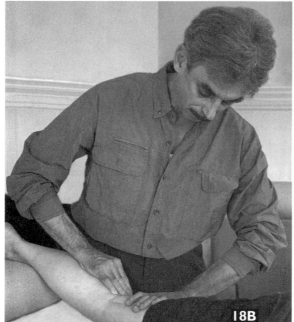

18B

The sensation of electrical activity is often a tingling, humming, or buzzing feeling of the current. The sensations I discern of magnetic activity in the tissue are somewhat similar, with more of a "pulling" quality. Magnetism is usually sensed as a slower movement/activity than the electricity in the area.

The normal electrical pattern of a tendon/ligament is experienced as predominately linear. This may correspond to their parallel fiber arrangement and adaptation to tensile forces. In comparison, the pattern of current through a visceral structure such as the stomach is more diffuse, with more of a rotational component.

In regard to the capacity of the human hand to detect a variety of electromagnetic frequencies, I have already mentioned the assertion of this aptitude by the researcher-clinicians Barral, Hunt, and Smith.[42, 74, 82]

Studies by researchers such as Motoyama, Reichmanis, and Becker demonstrate that the current of the acupuncture system through the points of the meridians has an electromagnetic component (see Chapter 2). Acupuncturists for many centuries have perceived the fluctuation of this current in their diagnosis and treatment. The acupuncturist-physician Joseph Helms states that acupuncture treatment activates electromagnetism in the body including localized ionic migration in the interstitial fluid as well as fascial and perineural semi-conduction throughout the body.[98] My experience is that as I detect the electrical current in a body area becoming more even and steady, the tissue exhibits relaxation of excessive tension and improved vascular flow.

This section on methods has included description of how these techniques can at times be combined for benefiting tendons and ligaments. My feeling is that while this can be quite valuable, it is not a substitute for learning one or more of the techniques thoroughly.

## Joint Gliding

A method of joint gliding can improve and restore articular health and function. Joint Gliding is a figure-eight pattern three-dimensional treatment approach combining direct and indirect actions. The technique has been developed over time in this author's practice and is primarily used for the joints of the upper and lower limbs as well as the joints of the cervical spine. It can be applied to costovertebral and all other synovial joints. The technique's strong grounding in a low-force approach is central to its benefit, allowing the therapist's continuous responsiveness to the body's signals and resulting precision.

The aim is to locate the optimal axes of motion of the joint and remove or reduce obstacles to free motion on those axes. The joint then has better tracking and balance in three dimensions. If there is hypomobility, the joint will have increased range. Joint gliding technique promotes reduced and more balanced pressures and pulls on the ligaments and tendons at the joint, influencing their improved condition.

## Assessment

First locate and assess the joint's range of motion and restriction. Look for the joint's motion barriers and their end-feel. You are looking for the elastic (passive motion) barrier, where all slack is taken out of the joint area tissues by the therapist. This is past the physiological barrier, which is the limit of the person's active motion at the joint and involves "muscle guarding"[138] (where reactive muscles limit joint motion).

Compare the joint's condition to its counterpart on the other side of the body and to other joints. Assessment includes muscular and fascial pulls in the joint area and adjacent regions, along with condition of the ligaments. Find which ligaments are more tight and which are more slack.

## Foundation Phase (First Phase)

a) Begin to improve the condition and balance of the joint's ligaments. Ligament work is alternate feeding-in and separating their ends, and other methods described earlier, including fiber alignment work. Ligament work (as well as fascial release of the area) will help to locate and reduce joint restrictions and identify intrinsic motion patterns of the joint structure.

The therapist can then follow the intrinsic paths of the tissues into their motion pattern (indirect technique). The joint will be moved to a point of ease which the therapist can hold until a release is felt. Similarly, you can use a Counterstrain positioning for the joint to relax the soft tissues and overactive afferent nerve signaling.

b) With the awareness of the joint's intrinsic motions including ligamentous balance, the therapist now moves the joint toward the motion barrier (which now may be considerably lessened). If the barrier is still significant the therapist continues to move the joint structure in oscillatory patterns going toward and contacting the motion barrier. Also use gentle stretch of the joint structure to challenge the restriction.

During all the motions the joint needs to be well supported by the therapist's hand and/or by resting the joint and adjacent structures on the table. Pillows or other props can enhance comfort and stability. Supporting the joint and the surrounding structure helps the patient to relax as much as possible. Support also aids in isolating the focus of movement to the joint itself, rather than a lot of movement of surrounding regions.

### Second Phase

Joint movement by the therapist will now include the joint motion barrier part of its overall range. The joint is moved rhythmically in figure-eight patterns which focus on its elastic barrier. Combine and intersperse smooth three-dimensional spiral-and-return movements with anterior-posterior and lateral-medial translation of the joint, as well as articular sidebending and rotation. Some distraction (traction) of the joint is often used.

The figure-eight movements combine both direct and indirect approach. The therapist's movements are always adjusting to the ongoing response of the tissues.

At this phase of Joint Gliding technique, both bones at the joint are being moved. Sometimes one bone is being moved more, and this can reverse. Move the bone in specific methods (described earlier in ligament work) to free the ligaments. A major goal of Joint Gliding is to restore, improve, and balance glide and arcing of the opposing joint surfaces. Sometimes there may be a click or pop when joint movement goes past the elastic barrier.

### Third Phase

If the joint's elastic barrier is still imposing a significant impediment to tracking and range of motion, this phase of Joint Gliding can bring additional release. The focus here is to move the joint through the elastic barrier to reduce its limitation of range. This change can be accomplished by one or more of the following:

a)   Support the joint and surrounding areas as well (done with a, b, and c of this phase). Find the position where all the slack of the tissues at the joint is taken up. After figure-eight movements at the joint's motion barrier, apply a very focused short-range stretch. This stretch can be a brisk movement but it is not sudden. Your aim is to "slide" one bone's joint surfaces on the other. The joint may go through the elastic barrier and may click.

b)   Gentle, oscillatory jiggling movement (often in a figure-eight pattern) is done while taking up all slack at the joint. The aim is to go through and reduce the elastic barrier. Movement is primarily a direct approach. In all three techniques here one bone is the primary mover. Usually, the other bone is mostly or completely stationary.

c)   Support the joint and take up all slack of its tissues, which can be done in a figure-eight pattern. Incorporate the sense of the pulls from the joint's ligaments to line it up at the motion barrier. Apply a small, direct, rapid low-force recoil-like movement to the elastic barrier. There may be a click or pop. The focus is to slide one joint surface on the other in the optimal arc of the joint's motion, which includes all three planes.

I use all three techniques for peripheral joints and only a and b for the cervical spine. A Counterstrain positioning can be an excellent starting point for proceeding to the joint's motion barrier and reducing it. When angles of positioning and movement are precise, little force or distance (short-range) of movement by the therapist can release restrictions and reestablish proper gliding of the joint. Thorough support for the joint throughout all the movement helps to minimize and eliminate strain on the tissues.

The therapist never forces a direct movement. If the resistance barrier still remains as a major obstacle you can go back to ligament work or to indirect movement. These methods may obtain release or prepare for a repeat of direct methods. Frequently you may find it useful to alternate direct and indirect approach.

Joint Gliding technique uses elements of all the techniques in this chapter. It was developed through ligament work as I searched for a more effective method to articulate joint surfaces and promote healthy motion of the whole joint complex. An element of the technique is similar to the joint play concept described by Mennell and illustrated by Greenman.[138] For joints where motion is largely limited by pain or there is instability or major inflammation, some of the elements of Joint Gliding must be modified. In these cases the indirect technique elements are more appropriate, with only cautious use of the direct methods.

To use the phase of this method with a focused direct movement at the joint barrier it is important to have knowledge and palpatory sense of the joint's ligaments and their force pattern, shape of articular surfaces, and axes of motion. Locating the exact optimal axes (arcs) for the joint's motion is a major key to the technique. For success with direct movements, the therapist must support the joint well and continuously monitor the balance of the fascial, muscular, and ligamentous elements of the joint region. Synchronize your movements of the joint with overall mechanical pulls in the body, electrical activity in the tissues, CRI, and breathing.

### *Example of Joint Gliding Technique for the Elbow*

The focus here is freeing the humero-ulnar joint of the right elbow. The goal is to improve motion of the bar-like trochlea of the humerus in the trochlear notch of the ulna, which can free both bones at the joint.

The patient lies supine with the shoulder area and arm resting fully on the table. The aim is to relax the whole area and minimize muscle guarding at the joint. Assessment by the therapist includes:

• Overall range and quality of joint motion. Find the active motion (physiologic) barrier and elastic barrier for the elbow.

• Fascial and muscular pulls at the joint.

- Elbow joint ligaments including the collateral ligaments and the annular ligament around the head of the radius. Which are tight, which are slack?

  - Comparison to the opposite (left) elbow and to other joints.

When the therapist finds significant limitation of the range of passive elbow joint motion (joint movement by the therapist), the following approach can be used. The main restriction in this illustration is of full elbow extension, with some sidebending and rotation.

### Foundation Phase

Options are:

- Fascial release methods for the elbow and surrounding regions.

- Use Counterstrain positioning(s) for the elbow area.

- Improve condition of the elbow ligaments.

If after these techniques, passive motion of the right elbow in extension still has much limitation, you can go to the following phase.

### Second Phase

Standing at the side of the table, the therapist's right hand grasps and supports under the subject's posterior right elbow with thumb on top. It is also the primary moving and listening hand. The therapist's left hand holds around the subject's right wrist, mostly under the dorsal side with thumb on top (palmar side). (See figure 19.) Include some support of the subject's hand. Your left hand at the wrist provides a long lever force for addressing the elbow. Both hands aim to isolate motion to the elbow rather than that of the surrounding regions.

By now the therapist is aware of the intrinsic pulls of the elbow area. Through this awareness you can find the optimal axis (arc) of the joint's motion. Incorporating those intrinsic pulls, both bones of the elbow are moved rhythmically in three-plane figure-eight patterns which focus on the joint's elastic barrier to movement. You are monitoring the end-feel at the barrier and the quality of joint motion.

Evaluate the movement of the trochlea of the humerus in the trochlear notch of the ulna.

**FIGURE 19**

Joint Gliding for the Elbow Joint. Balanced mobility of the trochlea in the trochlear notch of the ulna is a key element of healthy elbow function.

The figure-eight movement incorporates and alternates with lateral and medial translation of the joint as well as elbow side bending and rotation. Your right hand provides short-lever forces at the elbow and your left hand provides long-lever forces. The spiral-and-return movement includes both direct and indirect approach. There may be a click as the motion barrier reduces.

### Third Phase

If there is still a significant elbow joint restriction to full extension the therapist can use one or more of the three primarily direct techniques (see a, b, c) on the preceding pages. These are:

a)  Very focused short range stretch at the barrier.

b)  Oscillatory movement while taking up all slack at the joint.

c)  Apply a small, direct, rapid, recoil-like, low-force movement to the elastic barrier.

All three methods involve taking up all slack of the elbow's joint tissue and primarily moving one bone at the joint (humerus) on the other (ulna), which is stabilized. A central element is to locate and enhance joint motion on its optimal axis. Both bones of the joint are well supported throughout. Often there is a click or pop as the trochlea slides in the trochlear notch and goes through the barrier.

The therapist continuously monitors and responds to the balance of fascia, muscles, and ligaments of the elbow area. Synchronize your movements of the joint with body rhythms (CRI, breath) and larger regional pulls to the elbow.

The therapist's hand positions and actions for these three (a, b, c) methods are: **Right hand** supports both bones grasping under posterior right elbow. Monitors joint tissue and motion response. Is also the primary moving hand with a major aim of moving the distal humerus (trochlea) anterior in relation to the ulna. **Left hand** grasps the subject's wrist/hand area. Provides stability as the right hand moves joint. Helps position the trochlear notch. Often does mild distraction pull for the elbow. Often provides a lateral movement of the subject's proximal ulna by pushing wrist medially.

Elbow extension restrictions can frequently be improved by direct pressure to

- move the distal humerus anteriorly

- move both bones lateral-wards at the joint area

- apply some rotatory force at the joint toward supination/external rotation

- glide (slide) the trochlea fully in its notch. This is a main element of the method.

More complete, balanced range of elbow movement and joint tracking on the optimal axes would be the end result of Joint Gliding.

Never force a direct pressure in Joint Gliding. If full extension is still impeded, you can alternate with indirect techniques and ligament work. A common finding needing attention is fascial restrictions of the posterior distal triceps sheath next to the periosteum of the humerus, and of the fascia underneath the distal biceps and brachialis muscles.

Joint Gliding for the elbow uses both long and short-lever forces. I often use this combination for the shoulder, elbow, cervical spinal joints, and occasionally for the knee. While this can vary, I use primarily short-lever forces for the joints of the wrist and hand, foot joints, ankle, and sometimes at the knee.

By aiding smoothness, alignment, and integration of the soft tissues with articular motion, figure-eight Joint Gliding technique can reduce and balance pressures and pulls on the ligaments and tendons at the joint. The soft tissues no longer must strain to compensate for obstructed, inefficient joint motion.

## Essential Principles of the Techniques

There are some common essential principles of the techniques in this chapter. These principles are:

- Normalizing force patterns and reciprocal tension pulls in the body-—combined with precise attention to localized centers of dysfunction and stress.

- Harmonizing the peripheral structures (i.e. tendon/ligament) with the center of the body and CNS (through the vertebral column and cranium).

- Re-establishing movement that is balanced and unobstructed is basic to (structural) health.

- There are intrinsic movement and force patterns in the body (i.e. CRI and optimal fluid circulation). Facilitating these patterns to operate freely is beneficial.

- Encouraging self-correction in the body. This is founded on a belief in the intelligence of the body, down to its minute components. When given the opportunity, it is a self-correcting organism.

- Usage of small, well-targeted changes (e.g., at the foci of physiological patterns) can have a major impact when the clinician comprehends the overall structure and dynamic.

- Combination of direct and indirect approach, with extensive usage of indirect techniques, in which the therapist follows the body's structural and movement inclination.

## Comparison of My Therapeutic Model for Tendon/Ligament Injuries with Conventional Medical Treatment

This comparison for my approach is to the conservative care in the conventional model (standard physiotherapy and medication). I incorporate some aspects of the standard approach that are useful. The prevalent physiotherapy modalities that can be beneficial are heat/cold applications, stretching/strengthening exercise, electro-stimulation devices ("electro-stim"), ultrasound, and use of braces and splints. All these except electro-stim and ultrasound are used for home-care procedures by the subjects in the case studies. Occupational therapy can be beneficial in providing tools, mechanical aids, and retraining body usage patterns to minimize injury aggravation. Prescription and non-prescription anti-inflammatory drugs can accomplish temporary changes (in serious cases) that fit into a treatment program.

The standard medical treatment for tendons and ligaments seems to be quite useful in some less serious injuries, and has aspects that are useful in all levels of injury. However, in general it does not seem to be designed for actually reversing serious, chronic injuries with major tissue damage. As described in an earlier section of this chapter, the conceptual model it employs does not include much possibility of full recovery with conservative care, of that level of tendon/ligament injury.

While many physiotherapists have trained beyond the standard approach, the comparison to my model that I will be making here is to this most prevalent (standard) approach, which is received by the most patients. The various forms of heat/cold therapy, ultrasound, and electro-stimulation utilized in physiotherapy are all helpful for increasing circulation and oxygenation, reducing inflammation, and raising the metabolic rate of the tissue. These effects are not likely to be long-lasting in the absence of the following additional processes and changes: reduction of reciprocal tension pulls on the ligament involving body alignment patterns, normalization of neural activity, reduction of excessive misplaced cross-linkage, improvement of joint condition, and proper alignment of the fibers. These additional changes are promoted in my treatment.

Ultrasound is employed to lessen muscle tensions and increase circulation, and has some effect of reducing adhesions. Again, however, these changes are not as complete or long-lasting in the absence of reduction of excessive, inappropriate proprioceptor activity (this is essential in the muscle spindles—see Counterstrain description) for change in the muscle condition, and in the absence of thorough reduction of reciprocal tension (e.g., fascial) pulls on localized tissue adhesions. These additional crucial changes are accomplished with skilled manual therapy, which can also be considerably more precise and thorough in locating and treating adhesions (e.g., BMC, Fascial Release).

T.E.N.S. and other electro-stimulation devices can be used to reduce muscle spasm and alleviate pain, which reduces neural stress. Electro-stim (and ultrasound) can be helpful for inflammation when applied to cortisone or Ibuprofen cream on the skin, thereby delivering it to the tissue underneath (iontophoresis). The benefits of this modality are limited in their duration and their overall extent in similar ways to ultrasound and heat/cold therapy. The additional processes and changes (promoted by skilled manual therapy), which are needed for the other modalities, are also necessary for electro-stim to have more extensive and longer-lasting effects. In summary, the modalities of heat/cold therapy, ultrasound, and electro-stim are all useful in various ways, but on their own do not seem capable of accomplishing the major changes needed to reverse chronic and serious tendon/ligament injury. They can be employed as a part of an effective treatment for serious injury.

The stretching (active and passive) employed in physiotherapy can be useful to lessen muscular and fascial tensions, promote adequate extensibility of the tendon, and reduce adhesion. However, it is a very delicate and often problematic procedure to stretch a weakened, lax, and/or substantially torn tendon or ligament. As an integral part of rehabilitation, resistance exercises are important for improving strength and stability, and need to be used with the appropriate timing and level of exertion. Strengthening procedures are important but will allow a tendon to gain better tone only when it does not have too much tissue damage. Their improper use can increase existing neurological and fibrous imbalances in injured structures.

Common manual therapy procedures of standard physical therapy are massage, joint mobilization, and cross-fiber massage. These methods can promote some of the important beneficial changes for tendon/ligament recovery when the operator is very skilled. However, in general, the massage approach seems to be mostly focused on treating standard patterns of muscle groups and not on locating and addressing necessary changes in specific concentrations of fascial restriction and damage. Joint mobilization improves the mobility of the joint, but it can be problematic to use this degree of force in the area of an inflamed ligament with considerable tissue damage, which could cause exacerbation (indirect techniques, e.g., Counterstrain, would usually be more beneficial in this situation). The cross-fiber technique breaks down adhesion (depending on its orientation) but is often vigorous enough to cause irritation; it is often not very precise about bringing the fibers into proper alignment.

These standard manual physiotherapy procedures do not specifically effect strengthening and increasing the substance of a weak, lax structure (see BMC technique description). There is not as much attention paid to alignment patterns in the tissues in relation to the nervous system. In comparison with the osteopathic techniques that I use, the standard approach does not incorporate as much of a whole-body methodology that is needed to harmonize the periphery with the spine, CNS and other parts of the body core (e.g., cranial therapy), and to reduce more distant reciprocal tension pulls on the tendon/ligament (cranial therapy, Visceral Manipulation). Neurological imbalances such as inappropriate gamma-loop functioning are more directly addressed with Counterstrain technique.

In speaking about manual physiotherapy I am generalizing and describing the most prevalent situation. Many physical therapists have altered and expanded this approach, and employ a variety of in-depth techniques, including osteopathic methods. This comparison of my manual therapy treatment of tendons/ligaments is to the widely used physiotherapy in conventional medical treatment. The standard manual and machine-based techniques when employed appropriately can be useful components of an injury treatment program; but in the case of serious, chronic injury they seem to be limited in their capacity to specifically and directly effect longer-lasting, thorough benefit for the whole spectrum of processes and tissue changes described in Chapter 5.

There are distinct differences from the standard treatment in my manual therapy model. The relation of the model to structural/functional changes of recovery will also be described in Chapter 5 and seen in the case studies. It utilizes more of a whole-body approach. This incorporates a greater degree of attention to overall and regional alignment patterns and reduction of muscular and fascial pulls on the injured tendon/ligament. In general, I do more work to normalize the joints near the injured structure. There are manual methods for the injured tissue and its fibers including normalization of fibrous alignment, which are unusually specific (e.g., BMC and Fascial Release). The specific fiber and tissue work seems to be in greater detail. This directly addresses the problem of laxity and weakened, stringy, thin fibers, which receives little direct manual attention in other approaches. Counterstrain, Joint Gliding, Zero Balancing, and BMC methods are able to reduce inappropriate proprioceptor activity in and around the tendon/ligament and normalize segmental dysfunction, more specifically than the standard approach.

In general, my approach incorporates extensive usage of indirect techniques and is less forceful than some of the manual procedures of the conventional model (e.g., cross-fiber massage), which actually work with the localized area of injury. This low-force approach is useful for avoidance of exacerbating inflammation, irritation, and damage that can occur with overtreatment (including some exercise therapy) of structures that may be very fragile. Low-force work can successfully locate and address the neural and specific localized tissue anomalies and changes in small zones of a joint, ligament, or tendon (which can be small structures in total). This encourages an ongoing fine perception by the clinician during the treatment procedure, and thus can be more precise.

The therapeutic model I use includes a manual approach to a fine-tuning of the electromagnetic activity of the tissues (see "Techniques" section), which is not found in the standard approach. The electro-stim and T.E.N.S. unit do not appear to harmonize this activity in the same way. I also incorporate more attention through manual techniques to improving neural function of the ligament/tendon and its interconnections (including structural alignment patterns) locally and generally. As is illustrated in the case studies here, my model of manual therapy also differs from the standard medical model in that it incorporates the concept of a significant possibility for recovery from serious, chronic tendon/ligament injury with conservative care.

## Personal Background and Training

This description of personal background is intended to illustrate development of the skills, capabilities, and techniques involved in this therapy model for tendon/ligament injuries. It shows the gradual interweaving of various interests and methods to form my particular therapeutic approach.

Entry into this field grew out of physical activities of the high school and college years including various sports (baseball, tennis, and track), yoga, and dance. This led to an interest in learning about the body's structure and function. The impetus to an active life led to six years of employment after college in carpentry and farming, and ongoing participation (to the present) in running, weight training, and cycling. My learning about body function has been enhanced by study of t'ai ch'i and ballet (with Brynar Mehl).

Entry into the field was also stimulated by my interests (in college at C.C.N.Y., and post-college years) in the study of anatomy, sensing the body in a meditative practice, and the study of Chinese medicine. I will start here with my interest in Chinese medicine, which in 1970 led to the study of acupressure therapy with Kazuko Yamasaki, who had been trained in Japan. My study with her in Chico, California evolved into an apprenticeship lasting four and a half years. In 1973, I started a part-time private practice. Along with the techniques and theory, what I learned from Mrs. Yamasaki was valuable orientation as to the attitudes, way of life, and ethical sense of a health practitioner. In 1974 and 1975 I trained in shiatsu with Shizuko Yamamoto at the East-West Institute in New York and received a Certification in Acupressure Therapy in 1975.

From learning and practicing acupressure I gained a familiarity with the interrelation of a complex web of the entire organism, and familiarity with a sense of the electromagnetic activity of the body—both of which are useful in dealing with tendon/ligament injury. Acupressure (including some reflexology) was a major part of my practice for the first five years.

Sensing the body with a meditative focus began during my participation in yoga and free-form dance during college and post-college years, and was also part of more formal meditation after college. The practice of sensing is the application of awareness (full, active attention) to the perception of the sensations of one's body, including the subtleties of the internal proprioceptive and kinesthetic sense. This encompasses the perception of internal rhythms such as breath and pulse. My motivation here was curiosity and interest in the way the body functions and a desire to increase health and well-being.

Sensing includes a method of monitoring one's body sensations and identifying zones of tension or blockage, while allowing effortless, balanced motion of basic body rhythms (breath, blood flow) in those zones and their aligned, relaxed connection to adjacent areas and the whole body. Sensing evolved into an integral part of a comprehensive practice of ongoing moment-to-moment awareness that gradually became more and more central in my life; I have received expert guidance (1975 to 1990) from Lew Colburn, a former Jungian analyst who became an overall mentor to me. I learned from him that the body can be an instrument for reaching clear awareness and have continued to practice sensing up to the present. It has helped in the learning and application of the clinical methods.

Sensing the body along with the physical activities stimulated an interest in learning anatomy and kinesiology. I started independent study in 1970, which has been informed by the sensing practice, and utilized books, manuals, and journals. I began studying anatomy with Bonnie Bainbridge Cohen in 1974 (see below) and have continued learning this subject all along, finding it invaluable in my clinical work, and eventually teaching courses in it.

My interest in anatomy and kinesiology led me to begin studying with Bainbridge Cohen in 1974. In her teaching of experiential anatomy, cognitive learning is integrated with inner sensation, movement, sound, palpation, and imagery. The student gains an embodied understanding of the material, in part through direct (immediate) experience of his/her body. Body-Mind Centering includes the development of fine perceptions (of one's own body and that of others) such as the palpation of subtle tissue changes and detection of small shifts of movement quality that are so useful for manual therapy. There is study of each major body system (e.g., fluid, skeletal, organ), and its interrelation with the others in regards to alignment and movement patterns.

Bainbridge Cohen also teaches focused, effective techniques for tendon and ligament treatment that I have integrated into therapy practice, and has encouraged my interest in treating these injuries. Studies with her in 1974 and 1975 (and then at intervals up to 1995) had significant influence in the development of a clinical approach, in the direction of a more structural focus utilizing the principles of kinesiology. I completed the school's Practitioner Certification in the process (1985). Her example and instruction led to confidence that I could contact and beneficially affect even minute body structures in myself and in clinical practice.

In 1975 I started a manual therapy practice in the Bay Area. In 1976 and 1977 this was combined with part-time work doing acupressure with the chiropractic patients of Dr. George Casey in his office, gaining familiarity with chiropractic theory and practice management. Starting in 1977, I have maintained a full-time practice.

My interest in structural therapy led me to begin study of a derivative version of Counterstrain Technique in 1977 with an English osteopath. This began my involvement with Osteopathic manual therapy. I became certified as an instructor of this Counterstrain derivative in 1979, and started teaching courses. At that time I discovered Dr. Lawrence Jones' writings about his origination of Counterstrain, studied his manuals, and later took courses with him. His technique became a cornerstone of my practice. It helped with: sensing self-cor-rective forces in the body, utilizing an understanding of spinal mechan-ics, and realizing the efficacy of very gentle manual pressures to change the body structure. Dr. Jones' clarity of intention, economy of effort, and sense of humor have been a model to me as a health practitioner.

Another very experienced clinician who has been a role model is the osteopath and acupuncturist Fritz Smith, with whom I studied Zero Balancing in 1981 and 1982. Learning his method has helped the integration of structural therapy with acupressure. Along with Dr. Smith's technical expertise, his integrity and unpretentious approach to working with the whole person helped to deepen the efficacy of my work.

The osteopathic perspective was opening up for me, and the next component was Cranial Osteopathy. In 1982 I undertook the inde-pendent study of cranial anatomy, mechanics, and of the therapeutic techniques. This project was aided through guidance from a visiting Belgian osteopath, and from Paul Boudakian, a dentist who had received osteopathic training in Dr. Frymann's cranial courses. In 1986, I completed advanced cranial technique training with John Upledger, D.O., founder of Craniosacral Therapy at Upledger Institute. The Institute has made study of a number of osteopathic methods available to therapists in other professions.

During this period of cranial technique study I also received instruction from Richard MacDonald, D.O. and Jerry Slattery, D.O., and subsequently from Muriel Chapman, D.O., who, at that point in her eighties, influenced my sense of professional focus with her skilled simplicity and consistent deep attunement in her work.

The study and practice of osteopathic cranial work provided a more extensive sense of working with the interrelation of the muscu-loskeletal structure and the central nervous system—and a tactile appreciation of subtle tissue change and of subtle movements and body rhythms (CRI). It also incorporates Fascial Release techniques. As with all the methods I employ it utilizes a focus on the reciprocal forces and the patterns of the body, combined with precise attention to localized centers of dysfunction and stress.

In 1986, I began the study of osteopathic Visceral Manipulation with Jean-Pierre Barral, D.O., and then completed a progression of courses he taught. I found that working with the organs and internal body forces has been very beneficial for musculoskeletal problems. Dr. Barral's methods (which I have studied all along, and also taught) incorporate highly detailed knowledge of anatomy. They also include refinement of techniques for locating the centers of reciprocal tension patterns of the body, which are often the sources of dysfunction. I have been influenced by the scrupulous quality of his research as well as his clinical precision and emphasis on accuracy founded on confidence in the perceptual capacity of the human hand.

In 1985 I sustained a serious injury to my left triceps tendon, largely due to overzealous weightlifting exercise. There was significant tearing and then wasting of the fibers, and I was forced to stop my therapy practice for two months and then resume work gradually. During this time and over the next seven years, I underwent a number of different treatments (both standard and complementary) in a cycle of partial healing and re-injury from working. The tendon was assessed as being permanently damaged by two orthopedists (1986 and 1989) who advised surgical treatment with hope of only partial recovery. In 1992 I finally achieved close to complete recovery of the health of the tendon (90% to 95%) through a combination of strategies I'd already used, including osteopathic treatment-augmented by some intensive treatment of skilled Fascial Release, combined with the structural insights of Weslynn Hants, a medical intuitive. I gained an enhanced ability to work with these injuries in clients, including a sense of tissue health, precise alignment of fibers, and electromagnetic condition. Good health of the triceps tendon has continued and improved up to the present.

A Master's degree in biomechanics from Antioch University completed in 1996 enabled me to broaden the scientific and theoretical background for clinical work. This encompassed a range of subjects from the more standard curriculum to relevant physics, architecture, and muscle physiology. Connective tissue and its repair mechanism was a major emphasis of the program.

With my practice in its 29th year, many of my athletic interests and participation have continued. A major element of body focus is the physical/athletic demands of my therapy work. With sustained usage of arm, hand, upper body strength, and overall coordination and stamina, ongoing physical training makes it possible to continue this level of activity. In the last three years a Pilates-based program has been a major benefit that has also increased insight into various clinical issues.

My professional training has been enhanced by teaching trainings in osteopathic-derived structural therapy since 1979. These have been both independently organized courses, and courses through institutes such as: The School for Body-Mind Centering, the Upledger Institute which represents Dr. Barral's and Dr. Smith's U.S. courses (assisting with Barral's Visceral Manipulation), Authentic Movement Institute, and Axelsson's Institute (Stockholm).

Professional training in manual therapy has been founded on following my interest, and finding what is needed for successful results. This has led to timely instruction from expert teachers, clinical practice, and ongoing independent study. The combination has enabled crafting of a therapy model consisting of a blend of techniques, aptitudes, and principles. Its active use will be seen in the case accounts that follow.

# CHAPTER 4

# CASE STUDIES

The central focus of this chapter is case study reports from my clinical practice including a variety of sports, accident, and overuse injuries—and recovery strategies. Two in-depth case study reports are followed by ten shorter case reports, and then accounts of five recent cases. The first section is a discussion of the research design utilized to carry out my investigation of the benefits of manual therapy for tendon and ligament injuries. The case studies are a key component of this design. Readers may want this perspective on the rationale for, and the mechanism and validity of this style of research, or go directly to the case reports.

## Research Design and Methodology

My research includes a description and examination of the model of the therapeutic approach I am using (it combines several methods and certain skills), as it is employed in clinical situations, in order to determine its efficacy. The research data illustrates this therapeutic model and its usage. This data includes the presentation and analysis of case studies from my practice and also the relevant theory, scientific research findings, and other therapeutic models (standard medical) that have already been presented. The data involved in discussion of therapeutic and theoretical models is gathered from readings, interviews, and clinical experience.

A central component of this research study is the case studies. I use a protocol for the case study reports which Robert Yin calls linear-analytic and chronological.[89]

The data sources utilized in the case studies are:

• The thorough clinical notes I have taken during the course of treatment, which include the patients' reports of their condition, discussions with and reports from other clinicians who have treated the patient for the condition, and all the varied clinical findings I have made.

• Medical diagnosis of the condition, partially derived from X-rays and MRI findings.

• Discussions with the patients subsequent to the end of the course of treatment.

The criteria of therapeutic efficacy (variables) that I use are:

• range of motion of the joint(s) adjacent to the injury;

• findings as to the quality of the affected tissues, i.e., resiliency, tone;

• patient's capacity to function using the affected area;

• levels of comfort/pain.

The case study research design allows the incorporation of phenomenological methods that can translate nonverbal, perceived forms into articulate and precise descriptions.[90] I use both qualitative and quantitative methods in assessing the above-mentioned criteria of effectiveness.

A demonstration of the clinical skills I have developed in therapy work is relevant in substantiating the validity of the research findings, and also in construction of the therapeutic model I am using; so included as research data is a description of my training and relevant parts of my background/experience. A substantial degree of the accuracy of the research findings and efficacy of the therapy depends on a certain level of perceptual skill, so I have described how this has been developed over the course of my career.

Essential elements of this design are discussion of the standard medical approach to the treatment of tendons and ligaments and some pertinent theory and scientific research data. This places in context the clinical work described in the case studies. It is a basis to construct a therapeutic model and to establish the validity of my findings. The recent theoretic and scientific findings on the mechanism of connective tissue repair and healing are background for, and a component of, the therapeutic model that I am constructing.

The data will be analyzed as follows. The individual cases will be reported, and will be followed by a cross-case analysis in which significant features of the cases are compared and contrasted. Time-series analysis will be used at this point and in the individual case reports. This involves showing a progression over time of certain specific indicators (criteria) to establish causal relationships. Pattern matching is another form of analysis to be utilized. This method compares an empirically based pattern to a predicted one. Nonequivalent dependent variables are identified (i.e., resiliency of the connective tissue, range of motion of the joint) and matched to a predicted outcome of therapy to determine efficacy. If the patterns coincide, the results will strengthen the internal validity of the case study.

The research design is not intended to evaluate therapeutic efficacy through the use of statistical generalization (randomized sampling). However, another form of analysis I will use to determine efficacy is analytical generalization,[89] similar to analytical induction,[91] in which one generalizes a particular set of results (case study) to some broader theory/model. This uses replication logic, which implies that if one can replicate (reproduce) a similar finding by using the therapy model in other cases, it is a reliable one. This generalization has elements of a hypothetical/deductive approach, and will be combined with inductive analysis[92] that begins with specific empirical observations and builds toward a general pattern. This "discovery mode" is similar to Glaser's and Strauss's grounded theory[93] approach to theory-building.

Some of the rationale for this research design has been made in the preceding paragraphs. Here is a specific focus on this topic. Employing a case-study approach is appropriate when research is conducted in a real-life situation (i.e., my clinical practice) with a large number of variables and a context that cannot be tightly controlled. Because case studies examine people in or close to real situations and because they do not distort naturally occurring behavior through experimental manipulation and the creation of artificial conditions, they may offer better external validity than do controlled experiments.[89] Yin sees the case study approach as the preferred research strategy when "how" or "why" questions are being asked, both of which concern me in this situation.[89] In what Patton calls "purposeful sampling," certain cases are selected in order to find information-rich cases for study in depth.[92]

Further rationale for this design is that research with detailed cases affords the opportunity for a more thorough, in-depth investigation and understanding. I am using intensity sampling, with excellent cases having some typical qualities (not extremes) that are of sufficient intensity to elucidate the phenomena of interest. My case selection also has elements of what Patton calls critical case sampling, in which a case makes a point quite dramatically, "...if it [the therapy] works here, it can work in most instances."

I am a participant-observer in this research and while this has advantages, it makes it particularly important to strive for accuracy and to guard against bias. One benefit is that a participant-observer can discover things to which no one else has ever really paid attention, or had such good access. He can learn about things that subjects may be unwilling to discuss in an interview. It enables the evaluator to understand the context within which the program operates, and to access personal knowledge and direct experience as resources to aid in understanding and interpreting.[92]

Bias is a pitfall for any researcher, but the participant-observer must be particularly vigilant in watching for it. Here are some methods/approaches that I use to minimize bias. One tactic is to give the sense that my analysis has taken into account all the available evidence and that my information-gathering is thorough. I report and focus on the most essential and significant aspects of the case study. It is helpful to build a chain of evidence that allows a reader to follow the derivation of evidence over time.[89, 93]

The use of multiple sources of evidence minimizes bias and strengthens credibility, validity, and reliability. Using reports, medical diagnosis, letters, and patients' self-reports along with my own clinical findings that trace several variables is beneficial here. The use of multiple sources leads to triangulation in which converging lines of inquiry lead to the same conclusion, and thus strengthens credibility. In writing about case study research, Merriam describes methodological triangulation as the use of multiple methods of data collection (i.e., interviews, observations, physical evidence).[94] Bias is also minimized by comparison with the standard medical model (the predominant treatment mode in this society), thus adding perspective to my methods and analysis. Demonstrating my prior expert knowledge of the subject matter and clinical methods adds credence that my research is thorough, skilled, and relatively impartial.

In regard to the issue of bias as it relates to the professional (osteopathic) context in which much of this research is being done, it is assumed in my work that the professional integrity of the clinician would involve attempting to achieve the best result in any case (researched or not). So, the main issue as relates to bias would be accuracy and impartiality in assessment and reporting. Merriam says that one goal in case research is to have observations recorded systematically and with some detachment, a skill that I have practiced for a long time in recording clinical notes about clients. These notes are used extensively in the research.

Also in regard to bias and clarity, a potential pitfall for a participant-observer is to be so immersed that one is oblivious to the patterns in the situation[89, 92] Both the osteopathic and Body-Mind Centering methods that I practice are based on very rigorous, careful observation (assessment of oneself and others), and the recognition of patterns. This requires alertness and discipline-—and a certain level of impartiality.

The skilled clinician learns to monitor (evaluate) the effects he is having on the subject both through his intervention and attitude, which can change in the course of treatment. He is, in effect, part of the data (which can be reported), and the awareness of this is the skill of a good clinician, and of a good researcher. In this area, Patton asserts that conveying an understanding of the interaction between the evaluator and subject gives the study situational and interpersonal authenticity.[92] Discussion of the preceding factors illustrates how my professional skills and opportunities as a clinician are advantageous in the context of this research design and its implementation.

Research here includes studies of cases that are already completed. The response to concerns about this is that these are reports of thorough notes taken during the therapy and materials (e.g., MRI) that were done at that time. These were in-depth cases with systematic notes at each treatment session; I am not primarily relying on memories of past events. The cases are chosen because they are information-rich and very instructive. It is useful in employing post hoc studies that they be placed in context, such as how they fit into the overall population. Context is also established by discussing what factors are positive or negative indicators for success in the therapy (e.g., client's willingness) and how they obtained in these cases.

## Case Study A (Janet C.)

### HISTORY AND DIAGNOSTIC FINDINGS

Janet C., a forty-three-year-old university administrator, started treatment with me for problems with her right and left tendo-calcaneus. The right tendon was more problematic but she suffered from constant pain in both, and could walk only one block because of severe pain that resulted from any further walking. The subject reported that she had a high pain threshold, e.g., occasionally having dental fillings without anesthesia. The problem started one and a half years previous to this time. Janet said that her most severe pain occurred when attempting to walk after any interval of inactivity. This was most pronounced on awakening in the morning, when she experienced extreme stiffness of ankle movement for four or five minutes. The cause of the tendon injury was not apparent. Her office job involved mostly sitting.

She had consulted with an orthopedic surgeon and a podiatric surgeon specializing in sports medicine. An MRI showed the thickening of the right and left tendon sheaths and both nodules and defects in the right tendon. The right Achilles tendon sheath was thickened to three times its normal dimension. The podiatric surgeon said that he had only seen the level of severity of this type of serious Achilles tendon injury in marathon runners. Janet had a desk job and her primary form of exercise was walking. A test for rheumatoid arthritis proved negative. Her general health was good.

She had six weeks of physical therapy for the injury (three times weekly). This consisted of heat and cold applications, ultrasound, electro-stimulation, massage, whirlpool, and some stretching and strengthening exercises. There was also usage of heel lifts and longitudinal arch supports. There was no improvement from this treatment.

Previous to the physiotherapy, the orthopedist had prescribed various anti-inflammatory medications and administered bilateral cortisone injections. There was some relief but the effects disappeared within two weeks of completion.

During the whole period since the onset of the injury, Janet had weekly sessions with a massage therapist that also didn't appear to change the condition of the tendons. After physiotherapy she received treatment from a physician who administered acupuncture and homeopathic therapy.

Janet then consulted a podiatric surgeon whose examination revealed nodules and soft tissue masses in and around the tendons. His biomechanical evaluation revealed a modest pronation pattern. He found extreme limitation of movement, and administered injections of local anesthetic and homeopathic substances and a further course of anti-inflammatory medication. After a month, finding no appreciable improvement, he told Janet that he suspected some type of collagen disease and recommended surgery for both tendons to reduce the thickening of the tendon sheaths. She was advised that there was a possibility that the adhesions could return after surgery.

Janet was referred to me for treatment by her general practitioner and by the podiatrist, who suggested she try it for a month while he was away, with the prospect of surgery on his return. She was not very enthusiastic about the surgery, in part because there was confusion about the cause of the problem and a lack of assurance that the condition would not reoccur.

My initial examination confirmed the findings of the MRI report. I found extreme sensitivity to touch on both the right and left tendons with accompanying swelling and chronic inflammation. Her movements of the ankle areas were quite limited. I told Janet that the possibilities for recovery through the osteopathic therapy appeared to require probably six months, and possibly as much as eight or nine months of treatment. It seemed that her cooperation involving adequate rest, limitation of activity, and gradually increasing exercise would be essential for success. I suggested weekly treatments initially followed by less frequency as sufficient progress occurred. I would have a much clearer picture of the possibilities for success after three treatments. She said she wanted to avoid surgery, would cooperate with the resting and exercise, and was quite willing to begin treatment.

## COURSE OF TREATMENT

At the first session, Janet reported that she had continuous pain (most pronounced in the right leg) and could walk no more than one block before it became almost intolerable. Any dorsiflexion of her ankle was painful and its maximum range was 10°. Active plantar flexion was painful, particularly after 20°, and the toe raise was weak. I found that even the mildest touch of the actual tendon areas produced more pain. I found joint restrictions in the lower spine, knee, and the joints of both feet. There was swelling and inflammation of the tendon areas, which were noticeably thickened. The right leg was most problematic, particularly at an area on the medial aspect, two inches proximal to the tendon insertion. The tendon fibers exhibited some twisting and considerable inter-fiber adhesion.

At this first session I did Counterstrain positionings to free restrictions of the lower spine and of the foot (particularly the tarsal bones). There was also some Fascial Release work and ligament work for the joints of the foot. Specific treatment for the Achilles tendons consisted of induction and also separation of the fibers perpendicular to their length, in order to free the fibroses and adhesions. This was done using very mild pressures because of the degree of tenderness.

Janet reported at the second session, one week later, that she had some extra soreness after the first treatment that dissipated by the following day. I found that the left Achilles tendon was almost as sore to the touch as the right but not as problematic in terms of tissue irregularities or impaired mobility. The lower spine was somewhat more mobile.

**Figure 20**
Right Achilles tendon (tendocalcaneus), posterior and lateral views. It is primarily a blend of the soleus and gastrocnemius muscle tendons and is the thickest and strongest tendon in the body.

The electrical activity of the tendons had a jangled, uneven quality, and sense of "static." There were two noticeable areas of defect (tissue depression) in the right tendon: 1) a half inch from the calcaneal insertion on the lateral aspect 2) near the musculotendinous junction on the medial aspect. Each of these defects resulted from fibrous rupture of 35% to 40% of the total thickness of the tendon. I used some Visceral Manipulation techniques for freeing the lower abdominal/pelvic area. Fascial and Myofascial techniques were used to free restrictions and adhesions of the lower leg muscles and fascia including the tendon sheaths. There was pulsing in areas of the right tendon during the session, particularly during some induction methods.

At the third weekly session, Janet reported having slightly less pain upon awakening and noticed a little more flexibility. Walking was slightly easier although she was still not exercising. I found somewhat less edema and thickening of the right tendon and its sheath. With less overall swelling it became apparent that there was a spot on the medial side, two inches from the insertion, that was noticeably more thick and congested than its surroundings. The tendon fibers in general had a consistency that was brittle, stringy, and inelastic. As the right tendon was more problematic, reference from now on will be to this one except where otherwise noted. I worked with the knee joint and also with the proximal insertions of the calf muscles, using direct pressure on the Golgi tendon organs. There was also some use of techniques for freeing both ankle joints and the joints of the feet. It seemed particularly important to release fixation of the right cuboid bone. I used BMC techniques to improve the fluid movement through the tendon area (including mild pumping).

At the fourth session, two weeks later, Janet reported less stiffness and that the pain was no longer continuous. There was about one-third of the time when her legs were not painful. She was now walking three blocks at times, although this was still uncomfortable. I noticed less inflammation in both tendons and that the left side was less tender when palpated. Ankle dorsiflexion to 15° was possible although still painful. We agreed that there had been some improvement of her condition and that it seemed worthwhile to continue the treatments at one-week (and occasional two-week) intervals. I did some work to normalize the electrical and magnetic activity of the tendon and its surroundings. There was application of techniques to realign the tendon fibers, mostly from Body-Mind Centering, with additional use of induction. I used some Visceral Manipulation methods in the abdominal area with particular attention to right kidney mobility.

The following week, the report was that there was pain about one-half of the time, with the exception of stressful activities such as extended periods of standing. The tendon sheath was less swollen and enlarged, and there were fewer adhesions (better mobility) between the sheath and the tendon. It was easier to work directly with the tendon because of the reduced tissue congestion of its surroundings. Janet's lower spine was freer, but still had some restrictions that were addressed with Counterstrain and Zero Balancing methods. I used these methods to work with the spine in all sessions throughout the course of therapy. Findings of excessive tension in both hamstring muscle groups led to treatment of their insertion areas and other methods for increasing their resting length.

Janet reported one week later, at her sixth treatment, that the upper (proximal) part of the tendon seemed less sore and that she had less stiffness on awakening. Her legs mainly hurt while walking, and she was now up to six blocks. She started exercising with toe raises. There was more elasticity of most of the tendon, and its fibers were better aligned. I continued to do specific work with the fibers by alternation of feeding in the ends of the tendon together and then separating them apart (I refer to the musculotendinous junction as one end of the tendon). Adjustments of the skeletal structure of the foot proceeded more easily, and the improvements of mobility and alignment were lasting longer.

The session after a two-week interval was focused particularly on the tissue congestion in the tendon and on its electrical activity. Janet started to incorporate mild stretching exercises for the lower legs. Passive dorsiflexion up to 15° was only slightly painful. There was less inflammation and swelling of the tendon. The two areas of defect in the

**Figure 20A, 20B, 20C**
The technique here is feeding the ends of the Achilles tendon toward its center (20A, 20B), which can be alternated with drawing them apart (20C). This is directed toward realignment of its fibers and/or normalizing the tone and thickness of the tendon (see BMC techniques in Chapter 3). The tendon is placed here in a relaxed, slackened position with ankle plantar-flexion; this is particularly helpful to the feeding-in phase of the technique.

tendon (see report of second session) were not as noticeable, as the tissues were starting to fill in there. The fibers in those areas had less weakness, "stringiness," and laxity. I found that pulsation of the tendon area during treatment occurred more readily and that the blood flow through the area felt more full and even.

My findings the next week were that active plantarflexion of her ankle was painful only after 40° (50° is full range).[84, 85, 86] Janet said that she experienced some soreness in her calf muscles during walking. There was some soreness in the tendons proximal to her left knee. I did some work with both knee joints and with the tendons both proximal and distal to the knee. The techniques utilized for this were Counterstrain and direct fiber work with the knee area tendons. In addition, I applied Fascial Release methods to free fascia in and around the calf muscles. The area of congestion in the Achilles tendon two inches proximal to the insertion (see report of third session) was not as thick and had better elasticity. The tendon fiber alignment was closer to normal parallel arrangement.

**Figure 21**

Normalizing the fascias deep to the Achilles tendon. These include the tendon sheath and the periosteum of the tibia and fibula.

Janet reported two and a half months from starting therapy that she had only minor pain on awakening and starting to move. She was walking up to ten blocks with some pain toward the latter part of the walk. She could now dorsiflex up to 20° (full range) with the last 5° being painful.[84, 85, 86] Her calf muscles were getting stronger from exercise, including the toe raises. I found soreness during palpation in her feet and calf muscles. There was some realignment work done for the bones of the foot. Both cuboid bones still seemed to be prone to fixation. It was much easier now to work under the tendon (next to the bone) because there was much less thickening of the tendon sheath and of the fascia deep to the tendon.

The therapy was progressing well enough for me to recommend that treatments once a month would be sufficient. At the tenth session Janet reported that she was now wearing three-quarter-inch heels comfortably, and was concerned that she still had discomfort when she wore flat shoes. She was doing more walking and her toe raises were stronger. I found that the hamstring muscles were tight, had limited movement range, and needed a longer resting length. The tissue quality of the Achilles tendon was better in its elasticity and tone. I did some work with its musculotendinous junction. There was usage of acupressure techniques for the foot and leg to improve the electrical activity. Some BMC and induction methods were used to improve articulation and movement between the tibia and fibula.

The following month, Janet said that she had only minor pain with a few everyday movements. She could now walk one mile and would have pain only in the latter half of this. She was doing more stretching. I found that her left leg needed more attention and increased my focus on it in this session. The excessive fluid accumulation was gone from the right tendon area. There was very little thickening except for the medial area two inches proximal to insertion. I continued to work with the anterior tibio-fibular area.

When I saw Janet the next month, she was able to wear shoes with half-inch heels with comfort. This was five and a half months from starting therapy. Walking one mile was no longer painful. Her ankles had complete range of motion (both active and passive) with only slight pain at the end of dorsiflexion. Her lower spinal and sacroiliac joints now had significantly less restriction. This was also the case for the lower abdominal and pelvic visceral structures. The electrical and magnetic activity of the tendons seemed relatively normal. The two previous major areas of defect in the tendon tissue were no longer present. As I had done in all the sessions, I worked with the alignment and mobility of the bones of the feet. There was also application of techniques to fine-tune the alignment and mobility of the tendon fibers and their bundles. Regular therapy was no longer necessary, and I suggested to Janet that she keep me informed of her progress and call if there was any problem.

At a follow-up session five months later, Janet reported that she had been doing more walking, occasionally up to two miles. The only occurrence of mild pain was at the end of a longer walk. She had complete pain-free range of motion in the ankle joints and was quite comfortable wearing half-inch heels. I found some slight thickening of two places in the right tendon. Janet felt this may have been caused by some increased exercise on a recent vacation. I did some work to thin out these adhesions and found that the tendon tissue normalized quite easily.

### FOLLOW-UP AND COMMENTS

Janet was a cooperative client in her willingness to adjust her activity levels as recommended. She rested her legs and did walking, stretching, and strengthening exercises in accordance with my advice. Her attitude was good considering the discomfort she experienced, and she became increasingly optimistic as the course of treatment progressed.

After Janet's treatment was completed, the podiatric surgeon referred other patients with Achilles tendon problems to me. Janet reported to me that after an examination in the latter stages of my therapy with her, he remarked, "He did this with his hands?" When I saw him at a meeting two years later, he said good-naturedly, "You cost me a surgery."

One year after my last treatment, Janet was seen for another condition by the physician who had treated her tendon condition with acupuncture and homeopathy. She also had a session with a chiropractor she had seen in the early stage of the tendon injury. The Achilles tendons were examined by both these practitioners. They remarked on a major difference in the tendon condition-noticing the healthier tissue quality, lack of swelling and inflammation, and normal range of motion and function of the ankle joints. These changes had also been noticed by the podiatric surgeon in a follow-up examination.

When I interviewed her two years later, Janet reported that she had been surprised that the tendons recovered so quickly during my therapy with her. She has continued to be pain-free and her tendons have not caused her any limitation of walking distance since that time. She is able to go barefoot while walking in her house, and to comfortably wear shoes that have only one-third to quarter-inch heels.

## Case A Progression (Janet C.): Right Achilles Tendon

| PROGRESS | COMFORT/PAIN | CLINICAL FINDINGS/ TISSUE QUALITY | RANGE OF MOTION (PAIN-FREE) | FUNCTION | THERAPEUTIC TREATMENT/RESPONSE |
|---|---|---|---|---|---|
| Begin therapy | - pain is continuous; worst in a.m., on arising, and after any inactivity (right leg worst, but left leg also quite sore) | - more pain on slightest touch<br>- low back (spine) restricted<br>- S.I. joints tight<br>- knee joints tight<br>- joints of arch tight<br>- tendon is thickened, inflamed<br>- area 2 inches proximal to lower insertion (medial) is worst<br>- fibers twisted, stuck together | - any dorsiflexion from neutral is more painful, can't go more than 10°<br>- wears heels<br>- doesn't stretch anymore | - weakness of toe raise<br>- any walking very painful<br>- can walk one block before almost intolerable | - assessment<br>- work with spine<br>- work with foot, especially tarsal bones<br>- work with tendon, painful, thinning out adhesions around it |
| 1 week (from start) | | - electrical, sense of "static," jangled<br>- two areas of defect in tendon: ½ inch proximal to insertion (lateral side), and 4 inches proximal to insertion (medial side)<br>- left leg almost as sore to touch<br>- lower spine slightly looser | - active plantarflexion is painful, particularly after 20°<br>- normal maximum range-passive is 20° dorsiflexion, 50° plantarflexion | | - sore after session, but this dissipated by next day<br>- Fascial Release for leg muscles<br>- some pulsing in areas of right tendon during induction, then subsided<br>- work with lower abdomen |
| 2 weeks | - slightly less pain in a.m. than before | - spot on medial side, 2 inches from insertion, has major disruption of fibers<br>- slightly less thickening of tendon sheath<br>- slightly less swelling<br>- consistency of fibers is stringy, brittle, inelastic | - more flexible in a.m.<br>- dorsiflexion (slight) passive, is not quite as painful | - walking slightly easier<br>- still not exercising | - work with knee joint, proximal insertions of calf muscles<br>- techniques to improve fluid activity in tendon<br>- work with foot (realignment of ankle joint, cuboid fixated) |
| 4 weeks | - pain is now not continuous some periods not painful (about ⅓ of time) | - seems less inflamed<br>- left leg tendon is less tender to touch | - notices less stiffness in a.m., or after inactivity<br>- 15° dorsiflexion possible, still painful | - walking three blocks, some pain<br>- localized stretching still quite painful | - work to realign tendon fibers<br>- left leg responds well, pulsation during treatment<br>- visceral work, right kidney |

## Case A Progression (Janet C.): Right Achilles Tendon

| PROGRESS | COMFORT/PAIN | CLINICAL FINDINGS/TISSUE QUALITY | RANGE OF MOTION (PAIN-FREE) | FUNCTION | THERAPEUTIC TREATMENT/RESPONSE |
|---|---|---|---|---|---|
| 5 weeks (from start) | - pain now half of the time | - lower abdomen not as tight<br>- spine is freer<br>- hamstrings tight<br>- sheath is thinner<br>- adhesions are less between sheath and tendon | | | - work on hamstrings, insertions<br>- can work more easily on tendon because fewer adhesions around it<br>- work with lower spine (done in all sessions) |
| 6 weeks | - upper part of tendon "seems more sore" | - tendon fibers have better alignment<br>- better elasticity of most of tendon | - continues to have less stiffness in a.m. | - legs now hurt mainly when walking<br>- walking six blocks, some pain<br>- starts toe raises | - adjustments of foot skeletal structure are holding longer, easier response<br>- work with attachment of tendon on calcaneus |
| 8 weeks | - legs mainly hurt when walking | - electrical pattern of tendon seems more even<br>- less swelling, inflammation<br>- two areas of defect not as noticeable, starting to fill in, fibers not as lax | - passive dorsiflexion to 15° only slightly painful | - calf muscles weak<br>- start mild stretching of calf muscles | - pulsation of tendon areas happens more readily—blood flow feels more complete<br>- continuation of work to reduce congestion in the tendon |
| 9 weeks | | - soreness proximal to left knee in tendons<br>- spot 2 inches proximal to insertion is not as thick, more elastic | - active plantarflexion is only painful after 40° | - soreness in calf muscles when walking | - work with knee joint tendons proximal, distal to knee<br>- fascia around calf muscles<br>- alignment of tendon fibers is more normal<br>- work more easily under tendon (next to bone) |

# Case A Progression (Janet C.): Right Achilles Tendon

| PROGRESS | COMFORT/PAIN | CLINICAL FINDINGS/ TISSUE QUALITY | RANGE OF MOTION (PAIN-FREE) | FUNCTION | THERAPEUTIC TREATMENT/RESPONSE |
|---|---|---|---|---|---|
| 10 weeks (2 ½ months) | - only minor pain when awakening and moving | - feet sore, medial calf muscles sore<br>- significantly less thickening of sheath and fascia under tendon (next to bone) | - can dorsiflex to 20°, last 5° is painful | - toe raises starting to strengthen<br>- walks ten blocks, some pain | - realignment of bones of foot, cuboid still gets fixated |
| 14 weeks | - concerned with discomfort wearing flat shoes (is wearing ¾ inch heels) | - tight hamstrings<br>- tissue quality of tendon is better | - limited range (hamstrings) | - doing more walking<br>- toe raises stronger | - more work with musculo-tendinous junction<br>- work to articulate free movement of tibia from fibula<br>- acupressure techniques |
| 18 weeks | - little pain with movements | - left leg needs work<br>- swelling of right tendon is gone, thickening almost completely gone except for spot 2 inches proximal to insertion | | - walk one mile; pain only in latter half<br>- doing more stretching | - more work with anterior tibio-fubular area<br>- more work left leg |
| 22 weeks (5 months) | - can wear shoes with ½ inch heel | - electrical, magnetic qualities seem normal<br>- areas of defect not present | - complete (active, passive) range of motion<br>- very slight pain at end of dorsiflexion | - walk one mile without discomfort | - continue work with bones of foot (this being done in all sessions)<br>- work with inter-fiber mobility |
| 10 months (follow-up) | - slight pain with longer walks | - follow-up<br>- slight thickening returns after much more activity<br>- tissue quality is healthy | - complete range of motion<br>- can now comfortably wear shoes with only ½ inch heel | - has been walking more, occasional two mile walks | - thinning out fascia, responds well |

# Case Study B (Robert H.)

## HISTORY AND DIAGNOSTIC FINDINGS

Robert H., a forty-eight-year-old physical therapist, initially sought treatment from me for an injury to the ulnar collateral ligament of the metacarpophalangeal (MP) joint of his right thumb. Future references to "the ligament" in the case account are to this structure. Although the injury had occurred over six months before, he described his condition as very little improved, despite having had consistent treatment for it. The ligament was injured when he caught his thumb on the edge of a heavy table that was falling as he was moving some furniture. There was a sudden forceful stretch of his thumb away from his palm (later-alwards, and somewhat anterior).

Two weeks after the injury, he consulted an orthopedic surgeon (who did much of his practice with hand problems) who found a serious sprain of the ligament, estimating that 55% to 60% of its fibers were torn. An MRI had shown the tears of the ligament fibers and some damage to the postero-medial part of the MP joint capsule. The orthopedist found laxity of the ligament, inflammation and effusion of the joint, and a strain of the extensor tendons of the thumb. Compression and distraction elicited pain of the ligament and joint, as did flexion and any lateralwards pressure. Robert was given an option of surgical repair, which he declined, and was referred to physical therapy. My reports of the sessions with the orthopedist at this time (also five months later and during my treatment) are from the medical records and Robert's account.

Robert had started physical therapy one week after the injury, and the therapist's report at that time described swelling and inflammation of the joint and ligament. There was continuous aching of the area. There was pain with all the movement directions, as described above by the orthopedic surgeon. He found laxity of the ligament and evidence of a partial tear. Robert had ten sessions of physical therapy over a two and a half month period. The treatment was heat and cold, some electrical stimulation, ultrasound, massage of the hand muscles, and use of exercise and splints. Robert took a course of nonsteroidal anti-inflammatory medication (NSAIDs) for six weeks, and then at intervals after that.

Robert had returned to work two weeks after the injury, and found only minor improvement from the physical therapy. After that was completed he started treatment with a chiropractor who specializes in sports injuries. He had seven weekly treatments. The chiropractor's report at the last session describes thickening and stiffness of the ligament, along with laxity. He reports modest improvement during the initial treatments, then a plateau, and notes a tendency for reinjury from activity.

Robert was working half time, after being off work for one and a half weeks initially. He was doing one to two and a half hours of manual therapy daily (with some splinting of his thumb) and continued to feel pain and weakness with pressure and gripping with his right hand. Five months after the injury, he again saw the orthopedic surgeon, who found excess fluid in the MP joint along with inflammation. The ligament fibers still had some tearing, as well as thickening and scar tissue. There was still pain with compression, distraction, flexion of the MP joint, and abduction of the carpo-metacarpal joint. There was still strain of the extensor tendons of the thumb although somewhat less than in his first diagnosis. There was considerable laxity of the ligament. He recommended a repair surgery, and when Robert declined this he prescribed another course of physical therapy. The surgeon predicted that the surgery would strengthen the ligament and improve its functionality, but could possibly lead to ongoing adhesions and a problem with the MP joint.

There were five more physical therapy sessions with the same therapist over the next month. The report at the end of this sequence described essentially the same features as the orthopedist's last report. The MP joint and ligament were capable of very little motion without pain. It was reported that Robert was now getting only minimal response to treatment. There was a continuous aching in the ulnar collateral ligament/MP joint area. The anti-inflammatories reduced this somewhat, but there was no residual benefit when he stopped them. Robert had a setback from working shortly after this, and then started treatment with me.

## COURSE OF TREATMENT

At my initial examination I found Robert to be congenial, yet quite discouraged about the condition of his hand and his restricted usage of it. He did not want to have surgery but was considering it if his condition did not improve. At this point he was working half-time, was doing only one hour or less per day of manual therapy, and was avoiding handwriting as much as possible. Robert said that he had had some initial encouragement from his beginning treatments of the physical therapy and the chiropractic, but that the progress was not sustained. He found that whatever gains he made were easily reversed. There was constant aching of the ligament and the first MP joint.

Compression and distraction of the MP joint were painful. Any flexion of the MP joint was painful for the ligament, as was any of its medial axial rotation combined with abduction at the CM joint. There was some swelling of the joint area, particularly postero-medially. There was weakness and laxity of the ligament. Even very light touch of the joint/ligament elicited pain. The ligament had areas of stiffness and thickening and fibers adhering to each other, while some areas felt weak and overstretched. I felt one area in particular (closer to the proximal attachment) in which the fibers had poor continuity—they hadn't healed from the tear. The ligament fibers were not in parallel alignment and there were areas that felt "frayed." There was restriction and stiffness of the inter-carpal, carpo-metacarpal and radio-carpal joint areas, and a number of the intrinsic and extrinsic thumb muscles. The joints of the upper limb had significant restriction along with the fascia in the forearm and wrist. There were also restrictions in the cervical and upper thoracic spine, thoracic outlet, and thoracic and upper abdominal viscera.

I felt that the overall structural problems could benefit from osteo-pathic techniques, which would reduce excess stress on the ligament; there was significant potential for benefit from specific manual therapy work on the ligament and thumb. My sense was that recovery for the ligament would require consistent treatment along with conservative usage and exercise, and that if Robert was to proceed with my therapy, that he might achieve a substantial gain in functional usage of it in three months-—and hopefully close to complete recovery of function in six to nine months. I suggested three treatments (one a week) to start, to see if there was good enough response to warrant continuing the therapy. He was receptive to trying the therapy and agreed to mod-erate his activity with his right hand and do exercise as suggested. I felt that he had some useful exercise strategies already and that two of the splinting devices he had could be helpful.

At that initial session, I started some therapeutic techniques that I was to continue throughout the course of treatment. These were: clearing and thinning adhesions in the right ulnar collateral ligament of the first MP joint, and "feeding in" both ends of the ligament toward its center to encourage its knitting together. Both of these were done in combination with use of Counterstrain positioning for the medial part of the MP joint, which placed the ligament in the position of minimal stress (slackened). This had the immediate effect of increasing the fluid movement through the area, decreasing the swelling, and lowering the level of overexcitation of the localized tissue. I also did some

**Figure 22**
Ulnar collateral ligament of metacarphophalangeal (MP) joint of the thumb. The portion of the ligament that attaches on the first phalanx is more substantial than the portion attaching on the small sesamoid bone at the anterior (palmar) joint margin. Figure 13 (in Chapter 3) illustrates a therapy technique for this liga-ment.

Counterstrain techniques for restrictions of joints of the right wrist and CM joint of the thumb, and Counterstrain and Zero Balancing techniques for several of the cervical and thoracic spinal joints. In general the response was good.

I saw Robert for three more sessions at one-week intervals before decreasing the frequency to two-week intervals. At the second session I initiated some Fascial Release work to loosen rather stubborn tensions in the muscles of the right thumb, particularly the opponens pollicis, adductor pollicis, and the thumb extensors. There was some treatment for the cranial base and AO joint areas to encourage the balance and freedom of the entire spine and the dural membrane system. I did induction techniques for the thumb ligament and direct work with alignment of the ligament fibers where they were out of the normal parallel arrangement. The induction technique was directed particularly to an area of the ligament where there was still evidence of a tear (discontinuity of some fibers). This was about one-third of its distance from the attachment on the end of the first metacarpal bone. The response was some relaxation of the ligament (and its surrounding tissue) and a localized pulsation in the ligament area lasting about two minutes. Robert started some stretching at home for the forearm and wrist areas, and continued a moderate practice of some shoulder/neck and back stretches. He also did regular (three to five times per week) walking or stationary bicycling, which I encouraged him to continue.

The following week I found that mild compression of the MP joint was not as painful, and that he could do 5° to 10° slow flexion of the joint without pain in the ligament. He said that he was a little more comfortable on awakening in the morning, and that he found it somewhat easier to use the right thumb in his work of manual therapy. He was still using the thumb splint for this activity and was very cautious about using any thumb pressures. In this session I did some work to free restrictions of the upper abdominal organs and the pleura. I also worked with the thoracic outlet, and elbow and carpal joints. I worked to normalize the electrical quality of the ligament, in which I found a feeling of agitation and static. This resulted in a sense of more harmonious electrical activity in the localized tissues. The inflammation of the ligament and MP joint was somewhat reduced. Robert felt that he was getting some good result from the treatments. I agreed, and we decided to continue them.

At the fourth session, Robert said that handwriting was a little more comfortable, and that he was doing one and a half hours a day of manual therapy, mostly without the thumb splint. Swelling was lessened, I found less thickening in areas of the ligament, and the fibers were less clumped (adhered) together. His pain-free range of motion was increased (see chart) in MP joint flexion and CM joint abduction. I did some more specific work with the thumb joints and the fascia and muscles of the right forearm. The area of the torn ligament fibers was knitting together somewhat. In this session and others I used BMC techniques (including mild pumping) to improve fluid movement through the ligament and its surroundings.

We went to two-week intervals, and at the fifth session the ligament was less sensitive to touch. Robert said that it felt noticeably better after rest and particularly after two days of weekend rest (previously there was little or no improved comfort after rest). The inflammation was much lessened and the electromagnetic quality of the tissue more harmonious. I continued work with the cervical spine and cranial structure, using osteopathic cranial techniques. The cervical spine had better mobility but still was remaining restricted at the lower levels of C6 to T1. I did more work with the ligament fibers for their alignment, which was gradually improving. The small deposits I had found in the MP joint were reduced. He started resistance work with exercise putty for thumb and hand strengthening, which he had tried previously but was forced to discontinue because of pain. He was able to do some mild thumb pressure combined with medial axial rotation of the MP joint that was pain-free.

At the following session Robert reported lower levels of pain in the ligament, but that it was generally still stiff and sore on awakening in the morning. It was sore after working but recovered more quickly. He was now doing up to two hours a day of manual therapy on many days, taking a break in the middle. He could now flex the MP joint to 15° free of pain and abduct the first CM joint to 15° without hurting the MP collateral ligament. I continued many of the techniques I have previously described and specifically focused on the right wrist, in which the carpal bone joints and carpo-metacarpal joints were now maintaining better alignment but still needed better mobility. I found somewhat more strength in the thumb area, and that the ligament fibers had more integrity. There was slightly less laxity of the ligament.

He had up to 20° of pain-free flexion of the MP joint at the next treatment, which was two months from the start of therapy. The ligament had significantly less thickening, except in an area near the center of the previously torn fibers. Robert had increased his time of manual therapy and was able to use some moderate pressure (longitudinal compression) with his thumb in a neutral position without discomfort. I worked with the abdominal and thoracic viscera for mobility, and treated the thoracic outlet. My work with the ligament fibers was getting a more rapid response. They relaxed and realigned more readily and were less sensitive to touch. The result was more balanced magnetic pulls and a smooth electrical current.

At the following session I found that the ligament fibers were knitting together well, although there was still some laxity of the overall structure. There was no swelling of the area. The CM thumb joint still had some stiffness, and I did Counterstrain, induction, and specific tissue work with the joint, its capsule and ligaments. There were gains in joint mobility and localized tissue resiliency.

Three months from beginning therapy, Robert reported that the ligament pain was mostly after exertion, and that there was usually very little pain on waking. He was doing up to two and a half to three hours of manual therapy on some days. The MP joint pain-free range had increased to 30° of flexion. He was able to abduct the first CM joint to 25° without pain in the MP ligament and was using the thumb somewhat more while the CM joint was moderately abducted. The MP joint still had some restrictions and irritation of the postero-medial area of its capsule. It had almost no swelling and had some small deposits in it. I worked to ease pressures on the joint through induction and Counterstrain, and some fascial and muscle work near the joint. There was particular attention to the periosteum of the first digit and its interface with the ligament. The extensor tendons of the thumb were recovering nicely.

**Figure 23**
Counterstrain technique for MP joint of thumb. This positioning combines extension and adduction of the joint, and was used at several sessions. It places the ulnar collateral ligament in a relaxed state, which also facilitates other methods that were applied for its treatment.

There was significant focus on the overall spinal and cranial structure at the next session (now a three-week interval). I had given some attention to specific restrictions and overall balance of the whole spine in all the sessions, and in this one used more extensive concentration on some lumbar, sacral, and cervical restrictions. The ligament fibers still had some stiffness although their alignment was good. I did some work to restore resiliency. The electrical and magnetic sense of the ligament responded more rapidly and a smooth, steady currenting appeared during the treatment.

Robert reported three weeks later that he had increased his manual therapy work to three and a half hours usage on some days, and had experienced a little more soreness in the last week. The thumb muscles had developed some more tension since the last treatment, and he said that he hadn't done as much of the moderate stretching and heat/cold and relaxation strategies recently. I did some work with the thumb muscles and forearm fascia and muscles, as we agreed that the increased tension had contributed to discomfort of the ligament. The muscle work included origin and insertion-point pressures, and Myofascial Release. He could flex the MP joint to 40° without pain. The joint and ligament still had weakness, and I suggested he increase usage of the exercise putty for resistance work with the thumb and hand.

When I saw him next, the joint and overall ligament structure was stronger, including the localized tissue quality. There was some sense of electrical blockage in the ligament centered on the focal point of the previous tear. The work focused on increasing the integrity of the weak point in the ligament. I used techniques of feeding in the ends of the ligament toward center, alternated with very mild separations. There was also induction and focus on the normalization of electrical activity and magnetic pulls in this vulnerable zone. His carpal bone alignment and mobility were maintaining better condition and I continued to address this area.

At this time, the orthopedic surgeon examined Robert again. He found a great deal of overall improvement. There was no excess fluid in the MP joint. There was some laxity of the ligament. There was no pain from joint compression and slight pain from distraction. There was almost a normal range of pain-free motion (active and passive). He suggested that Robert continue his program, including more exercise for hand strengthening.

The last regularly scheduled session was three weeks later, five and a half months from starting therapy. I found that there was close to normal resiliency and elasticity of the ligament fibers. Robert reported that he felt pain usually only after a lot of usage and exertion, or if he stretched the ligament to extremes of its range while using thumb pressure. He worked full-time and was doing up to four and a half hours of manual therapy on some days, and in general doing as much as previous to his injury. He had 45° of pain-free flexion of the MP joint. I did some work with the fascia and muscles of the forearm. Also there was work with the much improved weak point of the ligament, and some fine-tuning of the fiber alignment. His cervical spine and thoracic outlet area were maintaining much better condition.

We made another appointment for six weeks that Robert had to cancel, and I then suggested that since he was feeling so good we could put off another session for a while unless he got into discomfort. I emphasized his keeping the hand and forearm muscles relaxed, particularly after days when he worked a lot.

Five months after his last treatment, Robert contacted me for a follow-up session to check his condition and do some fine-tuning. He reported that he was virtually pain-free in the ligament area. He was pain-free in the normal range of movement; 55° of first MP joint flexion and 40° to 45° CM joint abduction didn't bother the ligament.[95, 96, 97] He was working full-time, which was no problem as long as he monitored the hand and thumb muscles to make sure they didn't retain excessive tension. I found very little laxity of the ligament (about 5% to 7%). The ligament fibers had no thickening or adhesions except very slightly in the focal point of the injury. His overall upper body structure was in good condition. I did some spinal work and specific work with the ligament fibers to continue to improve the integrity in that focal point area. The overall resiliency of the MP joint and ligament was very good, as was the strength of the thumb and hand.

## FOLLOW-UP

Robert was examined again by the orthopedic surgeon three months after our follow-up session, and soon after also had an informal assessment from the physical therapist who had treated him. The differences they noticed in the ulnar collateral ligament were: lack of swelling and inflammation, normal pain-free range of motion of the first MP and CM joints, and a general healthy tissue quality and normal tone (almost no laxity) of the ligament.

I spoke with Robert one and a half years later. He was working full-time and was able to do as much manual therapy as previous to his injury. Handwriting and computer usage was no problem at all. He said that his usage of his right hand was fully normal. His positive experience with Counterstrain technique has led him to study and start to incorporate it into his practice. He said that although my treatments had been somewhat unfamiliar to him at first, he had been willing to continue them when he saw consistent improvement. His comparison with the other therapies he had tried was that they were less specific in their approach to the injured ligament, less comprehensive in overall structural approach, and at times caused more irritation. The ligament had even less laxity now (less than 5%).

I found Robert to be quite cooperative as a client. He was highly motivated to recover and regain use of his hand to return to regular work capacity. Robert moderated use of his hand and followed an exercise regime with consistency and intelligence. He had been surprised at first that he was getting as much benefit from the treatment, but as it progressed he increasingly had the sense that his thumb could fully recover.

# Case B Progression (Robert H.): Ulnar Collateral Ligament of First MP Joint (right)

| PROGRESS | COMFORT/PAIN | CLINICAL FINDINGS/ TISSUE QUALITY | RANGE OF MOTION (PAIN-FREE) | FUNCTION | THERAPEUTIC TREATMENT/RESPONSE |
|---|---|---|---|---|---|
| begin therapy | - constant aching that is increased from usage | Ligament of MP joint: <br> - adhesions in ulnar collateral ligament (areas of thickening) <br> - some laxity of ligament <br> - swelling, inflammation of MP joint <br> - inflammation of ligament <br> - feeling of electrical static <br> - restrictions of carpal joints and some areas of cervical, thoracic spine | - any flexion of MP joint is painful <br> - any medial axial rotation with CM joint abduction is painful For the lligament (active and passive) | - handwriting is painful to MP joint and ligament <br> - pressure with end of thumb causes pain (compression) <br> - using thumb to grip is painful, weak <br> - working one hour a day of manual therapy is painful; works using splint for thumb | - assessment <br> - work with clearing, thinning adhesions in ligament <br> - Counterstrain techniques for joints of thumb and wrist <br> - work with cervical, thoracic spine (Counterstrain) <br> - "feeding in" both ends of ligament toward center combined with Counterstrain for MP joint |
| 1 week (from start) | - pain is most noticeable at postero-medial part of MP joint | - tension in thumb muscles, opponens pollicis, adductor pollicis, extensors <br> - fascial and muscular tensions in forearm <br> - some areas of ligament seem "frayed," torn <br> - swelling, inflammation is most noticeable at postero-medial part of joint | - capable of mild hyperextension of MP joint, which is painful | - sense of weakness and pain of ligament, MP joint with axial rotation (medial) and abduction of CM joint <br> - stretching for forearm, wrist | - work with thumb muscles <br> - induction techniques for ligament <br> - work with alignment of ligament fibers—led to some relaxation, pulsing of ligament and MP joint <br> - work with AO joint, cranial bones, freedom of occipital and temporal areas of skull |
| 2 weeks | - easier to find some comfort after heat/cold | - small deposits in MP joint <br> - restrictions of mobility of upper abdominal organs <br> - inflammation is slightly reduced <br> - alignment of fibers shows some (more parallel) improvement | - mild compression not as painful <br> - first 5° to 10° of flexion all right if done slowly | - somewhat easier usage of thumb in manual therapy (uses braces/splint) <br> - stretching for moderate extension of CM joint | - work to improve mobility of upper abdominal organs <br> - elbow and carpal joints <br> - work with forearm, thumb fascia, muscles <br> - direct work with ligament <br> - work with extensor tendons of thumb <br> - techniques (BMC) to improve fluid movement through ligament area |

## Case B Progression (Robert H.): Ulnar Collateral Ligament of First MP Joint (right)

| PROGRESS | COMFORT/PAIN | CLINICAL FINDINGS/ TISSUE QUALITY | RANGE OF MOTION (PAIN-FREE) | FUNCTION | THERAPEUTIC TREATMENT/RESPONSE |
|---|---|---|---|---|---|
| 3 weeks (from start) | - ligament, joint still sore after working, but recovers more quickly<br>- still some pain in a.m. on awakening (stiffness) | - swelling is lessened (of MP joint)<br>- areas of thickening in ligament somewhat reduced (lessened)<br>- fibers much less adhered together<br>- areas of tear in ligament is knitting together | - more tolerance for CM joint abduction, MP distraction sill painful<br>- 10° flexion all right (not painful) | - handwriting somewhat less problematic<br>- working 1 hour/day manual therapy, not as painful<br>- now doing 1 ½ hours; some days, 2 hours<br>- now works without thumb splint | - work with CM joint of thumb<br>- work with thumb muscles, extensor tendons<br>- cervical spine and cranial structure<br>- work with ligaments, results in more harmonious electrical and magnetic sense of the tissue |
| 5 weeks | - ligament quality is now feeling better after rest<br>- noticeably better after weekends<br>- slightly less sensitive to touch in general | - electrical quality of ligament tissue is more harmonious<br>- cervical spine is somewhat restricted, but has better mobility than before<br>- deposits in joint are reduced<br>- inflammation is much less | - starting to do medial axial rotation with power putty (pressing), not painful if done gently | - start exercise of small circles with thumb<br>- most days, 1 ½ to 2 hours manual therapy<br>- start power putty exercise; had done this before, but had to stop because of pain | - reports feeling more optimistic about possibility of recovery<br>- continues to work with whole joint capsule<br>- alignment of ligament fibers<br>- work with fascia, muscles of forearm<br>- work with thoracic outlet, mobility of pleura |
| 7 weeks | - ligament, joint still sore after working, but recovers more quickly<br>- still some pain in a.m. on awakening (stiffness) | - somewhat more strength in thumb area<br>- ligament has more integrity (slightly less laxity)<br>- less tension in thumb muscles but still need relaxation<br>- wrist (carpal bone joints) and CM joint are maintaining better alignment—still need better mobility | - 15° flexion not painful<br>- 15° abduction of 1st CM joint not painful for collateral ligaments | - now using thumb splint mostly for handwriting and difficult tasks<br>- 2 hours/day manual therapy; after first hour, soaks thumb in warm water<br>- icing at end of day | - work with wrist alignment, mobility<br>- work with upper abdominal viscera<br>- work with muscles of thumb<br>- "feeding in" both ends of ligament toward center, alternate with stretching apart—combined with Counterstrain for MP joint |

## Case B Progression (Robert H.): Ulnar Collateral Ligament of First MP Joint (right)

| PROGRESS | COMFORT/PAIN | CLINICAL FINDINGS/ TISSUE QUALITY | RANGE OF MOTION (PAIN-FREE) | FUNCTION | THERAPEUTIC TREATMENT/RESPONSE |
|---|---|---|---|---|---|
| 9 weeks (from start) | - ligament is less sensitive to touch | - ligament has much less thickening, except in one area of previously torn fibers<br>- no swelling of ligament, joint | - starts stretching of thumb in abduction at CM joint, flexion of MP joint<br>- 20° abduction is pain-free | - still needs to loosen thumb muscles after working<br>- 2 ½ hours/day manual therapy, able to use some pressure (compression) through thumb | - work with thoracic outlet area<br>- work with upper abdominal organs for mobility |
| 11 weeks | - very little pain in ligament on waking<br>- longer intervals with no pain | - carpal joints maintaining good mobility, alignment<br>- ligament fibers are knitting together well, yet still some laxity | - 25° flexion is pain-free<br>- 20° abduction of 1st CM joint is pain-free for collateral ligament | - longitudinal pressure with thumb is all right if moderate, and thumb is close to neutral position | - work with CM joint of thumb—still has some stiffness, good response<br>- use of Counterstrain positionings for CM joint and for MP joint |
| 13 weeks | - pain is mostly after exertion | - ligament fibers are mostly in good alignment<br>- still some adhesions, but much less<br>- 1st MP joint is free of swelling, still has some stiffness, and a few small deposits | - 30° flexion is pain-free, active and passive | - some days 2 ½ to 3 hours/ day manual therapy<br>- is able to use thumb somewhat more when CM joint is in abduction | - work with joint capsule of CM joint, has some irritation of capsule at postero-medial area near collateral ligament<br>- freeing tensions in pleura and mediastinum |
| 16 weeks | - progressively less pain for regular, moderate usage | - ligament fibers still a bit stiff in some positions, although there is still some laxity | - 35° flexion is pain-free<br>- 30° abduction is 1st CM joint is pain-free for collateral ligament | - 3 to 3 ½ hours/day manual therapy<br>- able to do most manual activities if not pressured or stretched at extremes of range | - restoring resiliency to stiff portions of ligament fibers<br>- work with cervical, thoracic spine as well as lumbar and sacral |

## Case B Progression (Robert H.): Ulnar Collateral Ligament of First MP Joint (right)

| PROGRESS | COMFORT/PAIN | CLINICAL FINDINGS/ TISSUE QUALITY | RANGE OF MOTION (PAIN-FREE) | FUNCTION | THERAPEUTIC TREATMENT/RESPONSE |
|---|---|---|---|---|---|
| 19 weeks (from start) | - has gotten some more soreness in last week | - integrity of ligament fibers is better<br>- muscles of thumb have gotten tight since last treatment<br>- also, some forearm muscle tightness<br>- joint and ligament still has some weakness | - 40° flexion is pain-free | - 3 ½ hours/day manual therapy on some days<br>- handwriting not a problem if he takes enough breaks<br>- still avoids very heavy pressure on thumb | - work with thumb muscles<br>- work with fascia, muscles of forearm<br>- work with ligament fibers in central area of tear; electrical quality still obstructed, responds well |
| 22 weeks (5 months) | - occasional soreness after working, but not consistently to have blocked electrical, magnetic quality<br>- joint and ligament is feeling stronger (tissue quality) | - integrity of ligament fibers is better<br>- muscles of thumb have gotten tight since last treatment<br>- also, some forearm muscle tightness<br>- joint and ligament still has some weakness<br>- strength of some thumb area muscles is greater than others, need to balance | - 35° to 40° abduction of CM joints pain-free for collateral ligament | - using power putty more vigorously to build hand strength | - work with AO joint area and cranial structure<br>- work with carpal bone alignment, mobility<br>- work with ligament fiber alignment<br>- Counterstrain for the MP joint |
| 5 ½ months | - pain is felt mostly after much exertion/usage and if he stretches ligament to extremes of range | - better resiliency, elasticity of ligament fibers, close to normal<br>- carpal area is in good balance | - 45° flexion pain-free | - some days does 4 ½ hours manual therapy, which is the same as previous to injury<br>- still some caution of usage at extremes of range of motion<br>- back to full-time work | - work with center of ligament<br>- work with electrical, magnetic quality of fibers<br>- Fascial Release for fascia and muscles of forearm |
| 10 months (follow-up) | - in general, is pain-free | - very little laxity of ligament<br>- even center of ligament has only a very slight area of thickness, adhesion<br>- thoracic outlet, better mobility | - 55° flexion pain-free, which is normal<br>- 40° to 45° CM joint abduction (normal), is pain-free for collateral ligament | - working full-time<br>- must monitor had muscles to make sure they don't retain tension | - direct work with ligament fibers<br>- work with upper body joint mobility |

# Ten Capsule Case Study Reports

For these ten case studies I used the same procedures and research model that was employed for the two in-depth cases in the first section of this chapter. The reports here are done in less detail, and the reader may refer to the technique descriptions in Chapter 3 for more information on the manual therapy methods. These reports add breadth and scope for the topic, further illustrating the nature of tendon/ligament health and treatment—and the variety of clinical situations where my therapeutic model is applied to damage from sports or the workplace. All these cases involve serious and chronic ligament or tendon injury.

The case reports are:

1. **Extensor tendon of forearm muscles at lateral elbow (Alan R.)**

2. **Two wrist ligaments (ulnar collateral and pisohamate) (Linda A.)**

3. **Medial collateral ligament of knee (Alicia T.)**

4. **Conoid and trapezoid ligaments of medial shoulder area (Ray N.)**

5. **Flexor tendon of forearm muscles at medial elbow (Felix C.)**

6. **Achilles tendon (Kay S.)**

7. **Capsular ligament of spinal facet joint and spinal inter-transverse ligament (David B.)**

8. **Annular ligament of elbow (Felicia M.)**

9. **Distal hamstring tendon (biceps femoris) (Julia L.)**

10. **Hip joint ligaments (pubofemoral, iliofemoral) (Mary S.)**

1. EXTENSOR TENDON OF FOREARM MUSCLES AT LATERAL ELBOW

Alan R. is a 53-year-old sculptor, artist, and housepainter who consulted me for a one-and-a-half-year problem with his left arm. He first noticed discomfort after an incident of gripping and pulling to move some heavy cable. After two months of continued work the pain and stiffness increased despite his use of anti-inflammatories. Pain centered on the lateral epicondyle area of the elbow and spread into the forearm. He saw two orthopedists (one is a specialist in repetitive strain injury) who diagnosed an extensor tendinitis with substantial tearing. Alan limited his work and had various treatments including medication, physiotherapy, acupuncture, and chiropractic. There was occasional relief but no lasting improvement. Six months after the injury, one orthopedist suggested surgical repair of the tendon.

I found the tendon to be lax and weak, with misalignment of its fibers and significant adhesions. Supination and pronation were limited to about 70% of normal range and were painful after the halfway point of the motion range. Elbow extension was limited by 10°. Elbow flexion was painful in the last one-third of the range. Alan's wrist extensor muscles were weak and wrist flexion provoked pain after 40°.

At a series of four weekly sessions I addressed restrictions of his lower cervical spine, left thoracic outlet, left shoulder, upper thoracic spine, and costovertebral joints. I worked to improve limited mobility of the upper abdominal organs, particularly the splenic flexure of the colon. His carpal bone alignment and mobility needed improvement, as did restrictions of the interosseus membrane between the radius and ulna. Alan further limited his housepainting and more strenuous art tasks during this time.

During three bi-weekly sessions after that I continued to work with constrictions of the forearm near the elbow, including the periosteum of the proximal radius. Loosening tension of the lower biceps and brachialis muscles was also very helpful for the tendon. Full elbow extension returned and all movements were improving. I continued to use localized techniques to realign the tendon fibers, free its adhesions, and promote better tonus and decreased laxity.

In ensuing monthly sessions, the tendon appeared stronger and less "mushy." Four months after our initial session Alan was working about half-time, with very little pain. He used therabands for arm exercise. He noticed better coordination and fluidity of his arm usage. His pain-free range of motion was normal except for the last 10° of wrist flexion. I continued to work with the wrist flexor muscles and carpal joints to lessen constrictions and excessive tension.

After nine months from the start of treatment, Alan was working full-time and had completed a house-painting job that he had put off for a while. He was still careful with strenuous sculpting tasks and used his arm more in neutral positions when exerting much force. The tendon fibers had knit together well. The orthopedist examined Alan and found the area to be normal. We stopped the monthly sessions at that time and I did a "tune-up" session six months later, at which his arm was in good condition.

## 2. TWO WRIST LIGAMENTS (ULNAR COLLATERAL AND PISOHAMATE)

Linda A. is a 51-year-old nurse who injured her right arm and wrist in a bicycle accident. She consulted me ten months later, after orthopedic evaluation involving X-rays and MRI diagnosed a severe sprain of her wrist (involving significant ligament damage in the medial carpal area). The pain and instability was more pronounced on the ulnar side and involved much of the distal forearm. Linda had chiropractic, acupuncture, and treatment at a hand clinic. There was some initial improvement with each method, but no obvious benefit after that.

The MRI pointed to damage of the ulnar collateral ligament of the wrist and the neighboring pisohamate ligament on the wrist's palmar side. My initial findings were of inflammation, laxity, and fibrous disruption of those two ligaments. There was a nodule in each ligament amidst weakened fibers, indicating a poorly healed tear. Active and passive motions of Linda's wrist in all three planes were painful.

I began treatment of joint compression and anteriority (misalignment) of all the carpal bones, particularly the triquetrum and lunate. At five weekly sessions I addressed fixations of Linda's right thoracic outlet, shoulder, and elbow joints—and a marked tendency to ulnar deviation of the wrist. Her wrist movements became easier, with extension remaining most problematic. Linda continued to wear a wrist brace while working. The puffiness around the wrist was ended at this point.

At five bi-weekly sessions I continued localized techniques to realign the fibers of the two ligaments, while working to increase their tone and substance. The nodules were reducing nicely. There was still some pain at the end ranges of pronation and supination but she had regained a full range of motion for both. Linda was able to increase her computer usage at work if she used good ergonomic principles, but she still limited this to one and a half hours a day. She benefited by switching to a car with an automatic transmission. During this period she was increasing mild exercise for the arm and hand. The occupational therapist at the hand clinic told her she no longer needed to be seen there.

We continued treatments at three-week intervals. I worked with some restrictions in the flexor retinaculum of the wrist and the forearm fascias. A painful zone of her cervical spine became fully comfortable, and there was better flexibility of the cranial base. Six months after the start of treatment Linda had a full range of wrist extension and felt only a slight ache at the end of the range. She was still careful to use her arm and hand closer to neutral position when exerting much force. The tone of the pisohamate and ulnar collateral ligaments was close to normal.

Ten months after the start of treatment the ligaments had almost no laxity (about 5%) and Linda had regained full usage and mobility of her arm and hand. At a follow-up session the next year, the condition of the ligaments continued to be very good and the region free of pain.

## 3. MEDIAL COLLATERAL LIGAMENT OF KNEE

Alicia T. is a 37-year-old psychotherapist who had a serious injury of the medial collateral ligament of her right knee resulting from a fall while running on a hilly trail. MRI findings in evaluation by an orthopedist resulted in a diagnosis of a Grade III injury (substantial tearing, instability) to the ligament along with a moderate injury of the medial meniscus. After an initial period using a crutch, she continued to use a brace cast to immobilize the knee due to its instability. Alicia then had physiotherapy and acupuncture.

She consulted me ten months after the injury because she still had substantial knee pain and disability, and had seen little progress for several months. The knee was still unstable with motions such as turning to the opposite side. I worked to reduce swelling of Alicia's knee area and generalized irritation of the knee joint capsule. At five weekly sessions I focused on improving the alignment of the joint and increasing and balancing glide of the patella. There was some atrophy of the quadriceps, particularly its VMO portion. I treated the collateral ligament for zones of thickening, weakened "stringy" fibers, and fibrous misalignment. The inflammation of the ligament and the meniscus started to subside.

On my recommendation Alicia started Pilates exercise with an expert trainer. She had undergone surgery for endometriosis two years previously, and had developed low back pain afterward. I used Visceral Manipulation techniques to reduce abdominal and pelvic adhesions that were restricting the ascending colon, duodenum, and liver. The fixations in the trunk initiated pulls and force lines through the entire right leg, causing extra strain on the knee. Freeing these fixations was helpful to the leg.

At four bi-weekly sessions I addressed fixations of her lumbar, sacroiliac, foot, and ankle joints. Fascial Release techniques for the quadriceps, other leg muscles, and fascias further balanced the tissue pulls through the knee area, reducing stress on the collateral ligament. Three months after the start of treatment, Alicia could walk one mile comfortably on flat surfaces.

We continued sessions at three week intervals and the motion tests of her knee (anterior glide, tibial rotation) were much closer to normal. This was five and a half months after starting treatment. I was still treating the collateral ligament for a zone with some thickening and adhesion, but the ligament had regained 90% to 95% of its normal substance and tone.

Eight months after the start of treatment, the orthopedic surgeon found almost no laxity of the knee and said that the meniscus seemed to be fully healed. Alicia was comfortably walking up to two miles with some hills, and bicycling several times a week for up to one and a quarter hours. When I checked the knee six months afterward, the collateral ligament had only 5% laxity. Alicia said that she had resumed jogging and was pain free.

## 4. Conoid and Trapezoid Ligaments of Medial Shoulder

Ray N. is a 48-year-old industrial mechanic who injured his right shoulder falling onto the arm in a motorcycle accident. When I first saw him nine months afterward, he was working on a limited basis with pain and limitation in the shoulder area. Evaluation by an orthopedic surgeon pointed to acromioclavicular joint dislocation as the most serious component of the injury. He had five months of physiotherapy and received ongoing massage therapy. Range of motion of Ray's shoulder had increased somewhat, but the pain, weakness, and stiffness hadn't improved for two months. Another orthopedist offered the option of surgery to correct instability of the AC joint involving a Grade III injury of the conoid and trapezoid (coracoclavicular) ligaments—which are integral to the joint's stability.

When I first assessed Ray's shoulder situation I found his most problematic directions of (active) movement to be: abduction limited to 65° with pain after 40°, external rotation limited to 60° with pain after 40°, and extension limited to 35° with pain after 25°. There was inflammation of the major bursae of the shoulder and restriction due to fibrosity of the glenohumeral joint capsule. The conoid and trapezoid ligaments were still inflamed, with the trapezoid in worse condition, involving more discontinuity of its torn fibers. At four initial weekly sessions I used induction techniques to improve fibrous alignment in the ligaments and encourage knitting together of weakened portions. I began working to reduce adhesions of the shoulder joint capsule and to ease strain of the rotator cuff muscles and tendons. Counterstrain positionings helped to free fixations of the shoulder, upper thoracic spine and ribcage, and lower cervical spine.

Ray still did most of his work with his left hand, but his right shoulder mobility was improving nicely. At three bi-weekly sessions I addressed restrictions of his cranial base, upper pleura and its attachments, and all thoracic outlet structures including the subclavius muscle and sternoclavicular joint. Compressions of the wrist and elbow joints needed attention along with strain patterns of the upper arm muscles. Paresthesias of his right thumb and forearm were almost eliminated. He was doing exercises with therabands.

Ten weeks after starting treatment, we began sessions at monthly intervals. Work on the shoulder joint capsule had markedly improved overall joint mobility; and after two more months the inflammation of the bursae was greatly reduced. Localized techniques reduced adhesions of the two ligaments, adhesions of and a nodule in the previously torn region of the trapezoid. I had been working with a blocked, agitated electrical pattern in the ligaments, which was now more calm and balanced. The AC joint capsule was much more normal. At this point Ray was evaluated by the orthopedist, who measured his active shoulder motions at 90° of abduction, 75° of external rotation, and 45° of extension. Each motion was pain-free up to its final 10°. The AC joint still had 15% to 20% of instability.

Both mobility and stability continued to improve and eight months after the start of my treatment, Ray had normal range of shoulder motion. The coracoclavicular ligaments had knit together well and the AC joint was at only 5% to 8% instability. Strength was much better and he had returned to a regular work pattern. At a follow-up session the following year, the AC joint was even closer to full stability and his shoulder was at full strength and free of pain.

## 5.  FLEXOR TENDON OF FOREARM MUSCLES AT MEDIAL ELBOW

Felix C. is a 42-year-old acupressure therapist/teacher and fitness trainer. His acupressure work was usually four days a week, but had been limited by an injury to the flexor tendons of his right arm at the elbow. He noticed pain around the medial epicondyle after some months of strenuous rowing on a large lake. He had chiropractic and acupuncture treatment, and not finding much progress, he consulted an orthopedist. The orthopedist identified a torn portion of the tendon and prescribed physiotherapy. After three months of physiotherapy he ordered an MRI, which showed the elbow joint to be relatively normal, but showed a substantial tear in the tendon. Surgical repair was offered as an option.

It was about nine months from the onset of his discomfort when Felix first consulted me. At this point his acupressure work was at half of his normal schedule. There was some pain in proximal portions of his flexor carpi ulnaris, flexor carpi radialis, and pronator teres muscles. He had a normal range of elbow and wrist motion but had pain on passive motions of full elbow and wrist flexion, pronation, supination, and especially in the latter half of wrist extension. There was significant weakness of flexion and extension. At four weekly sessions I worked to reduce swelling of the tendon area and to improve the condition of a zone of the tendon tissue that had a palpable defect of one-half to two-thirds of a centimeter. It was important to employ techniques for reducing excessive tension in the forearm flexor muscles and the biceps and brachialis muscles, because all these patterns were contributing to undue strain on the injured tendon. Swelling of the tendon area subsided.

At three ensuing bi-weekly sessions I used techniques to improve alignment of the elbow and wrist joints. Felix's upper ribs, thoracic and cervical spine, cranial base and upper abdominal viscera had restrictions that I addressed. His forearm and elbow had a habitual pronation pull, causing a rotational twist that exacerbated irritation of the tendon. I freed restrictions deep to the triceps muscle. There were also important restrictions of the fascia and joint capsule over the coronoid process of the ulna. The tendon fibers were re-aligned and the defect was lessening. Felix increased his acupressure work 25%, which was fine as long as he maintained hand and forearm positions that were not too far from neutral position—especially when exerting much pressure.

We switched to three-week intervals, and after two more sessions, changed to monthly intervals. Four months after treatment had started, Felix was progressing well with moderate forearm and hand strengthening exercises. The excessive pronation pattern of his elbow and forearm had been normalized. During that time Felix saw the orthopedic surgeon, who was quite pleased with his progress.

Eight months after the start of treatment there were no adhesions in the flexor tendon excepting a slight nodule where the defect had healed. There was no longer pain over the medial epicondyle. Felix was working at 90% of his former schedule and doing moderate weight training. He continued to improve and was back to full work capacity when I saw him six months afterward.

6. ACHILLES TENDON

Kay S. is a 57-year-old owner of a real estate agency who consulted me ten months after a left Achilles tendon (tendo-calcaneus) injury. She noticed pain at the end of a European vacation during which she walked extensively in hilly areas. She was evaluated by an orthopedist and a podiatric surgeon. They both diagnosed a substantial tear of the tendon and inflammation of its sheath. She received two cortisone injections, physiotherapy, and acupuncture. When she first started treatment with me, she found all walking painful and was taking anti-inflammatories three times daily.

I found nodules in and around the tendon. There was a zone on its medial margin with a defect in the tissue and adhesions surrounding this spot. This was the site of most of the tearing which at that level was about 40% of the thickness of the tendon. Any dorsiflexion of the ankle was painful and its passive motions limited to 10°. There was considerable weakness in toe raises. At five weekly sessions, Fascial

Release techniques were utilized to reduce extensive thickening and adhesions in the tendon sheath. I used induction techniques to feed in the distal end of the tendon toward my contact with my other hand, which was condensing both ends of the gastrocnemius and soleus muscles-—in order to release tension in the muscles and tendon simultaneously. This technique affects the muscle spindles and the Golgi tendon organs. Non-force adjustments were used to free the lumbar, sacroiliac, and knee joints.

Kay was now able to do some relaxed swimming. She could walk five blocks with mild pain. At three bi-weekly sessions I worked with restrictions of both feet, especially the left cuboid and fifth metatarsal bones. The tendon fibers were being re-aligned, the sheath was thinning out and the area of defect in the tendon was filling in. Kay took anti-inflammatories only occasionally now.

We started sessions at one-month intervals, and four months after the beginning of treatment Kay could walk one mile, with mild pain developing only after the latter half of this activity. She was examined by the podiatric surgeon, who was quite pleased with her progress. The ankle had full dorsiflexion, with pain only in the last 50°. Plantarflexion was now normal in its range.

Seven months after the start of treatment, Kay was swimming and walking regularly. The tendon tissue was much more resilient and the adhesions of the sheath were greatly reduced. She could wear flat shoes comfortably at times when she wasn't doing a lot of walking or prolonged standing. Otherwise, a half-inch heel was adequate for comfort. These improvements had been sustained when I saw Kay one and a half years from the beginning of the sessions.

## 7. CAPSULAR LIGAMENT OF SPINAL FACET JOINT AND SPINAL INTERTRANSVERSE LIGAMENT

Daniel B. is a 38-year-old business executive who is co-owner of a consulting firm. He injured his left lower back fourteen months prior to consulting me. A windsurfing accident involved a sudden forceful twist to his trunk and a fall. MRI findings and exams by two orthopedic surgeons and a physiotherapist revealed a mild disc bulge at L4-5 and a 5 mm gap of the left zygapophyseal (articular facet) joint of L4-5. The corresponding joint on the right had a 1.5 mm gap. They found instability of his joint and symptoms of a left L5 radiculopathy. Daniel had pain from sitting, standing, bending, and walking. There was some weakness of lower limb muscles, and pain and paresthesia in his left foot. One orthopedist recommended surgery.

Daniel chose to try a conservative care approach and was treated with non-steroidal anti-inflammatories (NSAIDS) and two epidural steroidal blocks. He had chiropractic care and four months of physiotherapy. Improvement from these approaches was not sustained.

I found limitation of lumbar lateral bending and stiffness of the lower thoracic spine. Counterstrain techniques treated the lower thoracic, lumbar, and sacroiliac joints. Fascial Release was helpful for addressing the paraspinal, gluteal, and hip areas. At six weekly sessions I employed BMC techniques of feeding in the capsular ligaments of the left L4-5 articular facet joint and the L4-5 intertransverse ligament (which was "stringy" and twisted). The goal here was to reduce instability of this spinal segment involving laxity of these two ligaments. I also worked to lessen stiffness and adhesions in the left iliolumbar ligament.

Daniel still avoided prolonged sitting when possible and continued exercise instruction from the physiotherapist, gradually adding some swimming and recumbent stationary bicycling. The weekly sessions were followed by eight bi-weekly sessions during which I continued localized work with the facet capsule and other L4-5 ligaments including the ligamentum flavum. I used manual contact with the vertebrae and leverage from the ribs and pelvis to direct forces into the localized zones of the ligaments. Techniques were also employed to harmonize the Cranial Rhythmic Impulse through the lower spine and lower limbs. After four months of the osteopathic treatment, Daniel's leg and foot symptoms were reduced except after substantial activity.

The orthopedist found no muscle weakness. The left facet joint felt more stable with motion testing.

After six months of treatment the intertransverse ligament and the facet joint capsule felt normal to me in terms of their tonus, resiliency, and stability. The left side of the joint was better positioned and more stable. Pain and nerve symptoms were markedly reduced and confined to the low back area. At this point we continued sessions at three-week intervals. The L4-5 ligaments continued to be normal one year from the start of treatment, and his overall functioning was about 85% to 90% of his previous level.

## 8. ANNULAR LIGAMENT OF ELBOW

Felicia M. is a 45-year-old music teacher/pianist who had right arm and wrist pain resulting from a poorly set fracture of the head of the radius, fifteen years earlier. At a recent examination by an orthopedic surgeon involving X-rays, he diagnosed an enlargement of the radial head along with inferior displacement. He found some arthritic change of the elbow joint. All of Felicia's right elbow movements were stiff and limited. Pronation, supination, and extension were limited to about 20° less than normal, and elbow flexion was restricted by 25°. In the years since the fracture, she had been treated with acupuncture, chiropractic, and physiotherapy.

I found a major problem with the annular ligament that holds the radial head in place by wrapping around it and attaching to the ulna. The inferior displacement of the radial head had contributed to the ligament's tearing and its subsequent thickening, adhesions, inelasticity, and disorganized fibrous alignment. Soreness of the ligament was a component of Felicia's elbow pain, which could be provoked by movements in any direction. We commenced weekly sessions at which I addressed the specific tissue condition of the annular ligament along with restrictions of the thoracic outlet, cervical spine, and thoracic spine; all these were involved in a right rotation of her thorax.

Felicia limited her piano playing to one hour per day at this point and minimized her computer usage, which was also an irritant to the arm. At five weekly sessions I worked with constriction of both collateral ligaments of the elbow and some adhesions in other parts of the joint capsule. The elbow problem seemed to have a significant emotional component that surfaced during the initial sessions. It required some re-adjustment for Felicia to accept the increasing mobility of her arm after fifteen years.

At three bi-weekly sessions I noticed that the four major elbow motions had increased in range to about 10° below normal range. The fascias and muscles of the arm were treated for restrictions along with significant attention to re-alignment of the carpal joints. Felicia started instruction to promote more balanced arm and hand usage in piano playing and computer work. A discordant electrical pattern ("static") of the annular ligament tissue had been normalized, and its tissue was gaining resiliency and pliability. Both attachments of the ligament on the ulna were condensing slightly as I worked to normalize position of the radial head.

After four sessions at monthly intervals (seven months from the start of treatment) Felicia had full and much smoother pain-free elbow motion in all four directions. She played the piano up to two hours a day and could use the computer as needed without pain.

She returned for another session after four months and had a slight decrease in her range of elbow extension and some stiffness of the ligament. This responded well to treatment and her comfort level has been good for one year. The enlarged radial head was now positioned more normally. The progression of this case was somewhat slower and the subsequent results affected by the fairly difficult emotional elements associated with Felicia's elbow problem. At times she would discontinue exercising the arm and some stiffness returned. However, she would return for a "tune-up" session and start exercising, and the elbow was back to normal function.

## 9. DISTAL HAMSTRING (BICEPS FEMORIS) TENDON

This is the case that was reported on the second page of Chapter 1. Julia L. is a dancer and co-chair of a dance department at a university. The case report depicts the obstacles she faced, the therapy process for her injury, and her gradual recovery.

## 10. HIP JOINT LIGAMENTS (PUBOFEMORAL, ILIOFEMORAL)

Mary S. is a 45-year-old dance teacher who was very limited by a right hip injury that had occurred several months before I first saw her. She traced the hip pain and limitation to three sessions of strenuous dance movement when she was quite fatigued and cold. At the time she was recovering from a left knee injury that caused her to put more weight onto her right leg. She had chiropractic treatment and then consulted an orthopedist. X-rays of the area revealed a normal hip joint. He suspected iliopectineal bursitis (in the anterior hip region), prescribed anti-inflammatory medication, and referred her to physiotherapy. She was treated for two months and initially had some improvement, but it wasn't sustained after that. She then had massage and acupuncture treatment. At this point walking for more than five to ten minutes was quite uncomfortable.

At Mary's first session I found marked resistance to adduction and external rotation of her femur. All hip joint movements were stiff and provoked pain toward the end range of movement. On palpation I found zones of the anterior hip capsule ligaments (pubofemoral and the medial part of the iliofemoral) that were stringy, swollen, had disorganized fibers, and contained some nodules. The tearing in these ligaments had left zones with discontinuity of the fibers, which showed significant weakening. The posterior capsular ligaments (ischiofemoral and lateral iliofemoral) were very tight and overly fibrous. I used induction and BMC techniques to realign the fibers, release adhesions, and reduce tissue irritation. At four weekly sessions work was also directed to freeing and balancing the sacroiliac, sacrococcygeal, and lumbar spinal joints, and the pubic symphysis. Mary could move more easily and now found gentle stretching more useful.

At the following three bi-weekly sessions I continued to use osteo-pathic visceral manipulation to free restrictions and improve mobility in the right pleura, duodenum, bladder, cecum, restrictions in , and right kidney. This work contributed to releasing tension in the psoas muscle. Excessive tensions in the piriformis, both obturators, quadri-ceps, and adductor muscles also received attention. The ischiofemoral ligament was more pliable and the damaged portions of the pub-ofemoral and medial iliofemoral ligaments were knitting together, gaining better tone, and were better organized. At the end of this series Mary could walk a half mile on flat ground fairly comfortably. All hip movements were better in range, with the end ranges of adduction and internal rotation continuing to have some restriction and pain. Mary started Pilates exercise with an expert trainer.

We then met for three sessions at which I continued localized work with the hip ligaments and Fascial Release techniques for the thigh, gluteal, and hip rotator muscles. It was helpful to balance the foot, knee, lumbar, and lower thoracic joints. Five months after the start of treatments Mary could walk one and a quarter miles comfort-ably and was demonstrating more of the movements for her dance students. All hip movements were normal except for the last 5° of adduction. At a follow-up session (eight months from the start) she had normal strength of her hip muscles and the tissue quality of the ligaments was healthy. When I spoke with her the following year, Mary said that she had returned to her previous dance workouts and was free of pain.

## Five Recent Cases

Each of these further accounts for tendons and ligaments (new to the book's second edition) illustrates additional elements of sports and overuse injury and recovery, using the author's treatment model.

**Case 11** recounts how the methods for treating chronically injured elbow ligaments affect Anna's serious nerve injury following a skating accident.

The central element of **Case 12** describes James' therapy for the rotator cuff of the shoulder, one of the most widespread tendon injuries in sports, accidents, and overuse/repetitive strain.

**Case 13** highlights treatment of badly damaged ligaments in Daniel's major, chronic acromio-clavicular joint dislocation-a condition that rarely resolves with conservative care.

The account of a patellar ligament problem of Greg's knee in **Case 14** portrays the approach to a frequent injury in basketball and other sports. It gives a clear example of a tissue degeneration injury in a ligament, and offers strategies for recovery.

**Case 15** involves what is perhaps the most frequent ligament injury, sprain of the lateral ankle. An important element of Maria's therapy is how it includes her return to dance and running.

In the book's 12 cases up to this point, exercise has been an essential factor in the person's recovery. For these five cases, particularly **Case 14** on the knee's patellar ligament, I have included more detail on the role of exercise synchronized with manual therapy techniques.

### 11. Ulnar Collateral Ligament of Elbow (Distal Triceps Tendon) (Ulnar Nerve)

Anna L. is a 56-year-old physician who consulted me three months after falling backward while ice-skating. She landed fully on her right elbow, fracturing the olecranon of the ulna into four pieces. One piece was shattered and displaced and remained jutting out into the joint margin, as the surgeon was unable to place it properly. Two pins and wire were placed to fixate the bone and joint. One of the pins had slipped and bent, preventing full elbow extension following the cast removal after four weeks. The pins had been removed the week I saw her.

Anna had physiotherapy three times a week after the cast removal. Treatment was iontophoresis (with electro-stim), massage, and passive range of motion exercises done by the therapist. Three weeks before contacting me, immediately after vigorous passive stretching for elbow flexion in therapy, she developed constant numbness and cold in her fourth and fifth fingers and palm. Her orthopedist and a neurosurgeon diagnosed ulnar nerve injury at the elbow. They recommended a surgical procedure to free the nerve.

I found Anna to be cooperative, although she was puzzled by the deterioration of her arm condition after having been diligent in following the exercise and treatment prescribed for her. She had acute soreness at her medial elbow and posteriorly at the distal triceps tendon where the wire for the pin had been exerting pressure. The triceps tendon had a divot at the spot where the wire had dug into it, and was flaccid and swollen overall.

Supination and pronation caused pain at the medial elbow. Her passive elbow flexion was about 130° and passive extension about 15° short of straight. She had weakness of fifth finger adduction and thumb pinching as ulnar nerve signs.

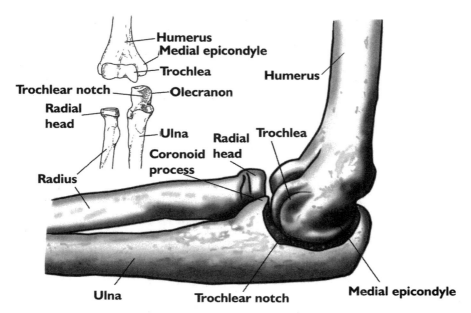

**Figure 23A**
Elbow joint, medial view. The ulnar (medial) collateral ligament of the joint extends in a fan shape from the medial epicondyle of the humerus to the ulna below the trochlear notch and to the coronoid process.

Treatment at the first of two bi-monthly sessions addressed adhesions at the triceps attachment on the ulna, congestion under the triceps proximal to the elbow, tightness of the forearm (wrist) flexor muscle, adhesions of the anterior elbow joint capsule. The medial (ulnar) collateral elbow ligament was swollen, inelastic and somewhat rigid, with disorganized fiber alignment and accumulation of waste material in its tissue.

Anna had nerve conduction studies that showed major deficits in ulnar nerve function. The physician administering the test told her that her measurements were an obvious, clear indication for surgery without delay. She had marked weakness in thumb pinching and other hand usage. Muscle wasting in her hand was apparent. She consulted the leading neurologist for hand injuries in her area, who also recommended surgical decompression. He felt she was risking permanent damage. The surgery was scheduled for one month away.

Because she now felt less pain and movement restriction, Anna wanted to continue treatment, and she had four weekly sessions preceding the surgery. Techniques focused on freeing her upper ribs, thoracic outlet, cervical and upper thoracic spine, and cranial base. Her right pleura and upper abdominal viscera received attention for restrictions. I loosened adhesions in and under the distal right brachialis and biceps muscles.

Counterstrain and Joint Gliding techniques at the elbow were used to improve humero-ulnar and radial head alignment and mobility. Her ulnar collateral ligament was regaining pliability, with less adhesion, and cleaner, more streamlined condition of its tissue composition. At the third weekly session, Anna's elbow could be extended fully with passive motion. I worked to free the ulnar nerve at the elbow where it passes under the medial collateral ligament between the medial epicondyle and olecranon. At the fourth weekly session (sixth overall) she reported more hand and arm strength and greater sensation in her right palm.

Surgery was now planned for her return from a 12-day vacation in the Alps. She scheduled another treatment for the day before the surgery, immediately on her return from Europe. At that session Anna said that the numbness had receded to only the anterior side of her fourth and fifth fingers; the palm was clear. Her muscles were much stronger and handwriting was now normal.

She contacted the surgeon, who decided to examine her before any surgery. He found normal strength of her right hand lumbrical muscles (indicators of ulnar nerve function) and normal sensation at her fourth and fifth fingertip. Surgery was postponed indefinitely.

Anna had three more sessions at three-week intervals in which I continued to normalize her medial collateral ligament and right elbow joint. Her upper arm fascia still needed attention for congestion. The only remaining pain was at the distal triceps tendon attachment. The defect in her tendon was reduced and I worked to clear it of excess fluid and waste material, and to promote better tone and strength. Elbow flexion and extension were normal. The numbness was now infrequent and only a "shadow" when it occurred.

One and a half years later Anna has normal strength, function, mobility and sensation of her right elbow and hand. She is active in weight training, hiking, yoga, and ice-skating.

## 12. Supraspinatus Tendon, Biceps Tendon (Rotator Cuff of Shoulder)

James G. is a leading classical pianist. For 25 years he has played a year-round schedule throughout the U.S., Europe, and Asia. A large, energetic man of 52, he injured his left shoulder on tour as he lifted a suitcase in the airport. He continued his concert dates but felt increasing discomfort. X-rays showed a bone spur on the acromion affecting the upper rotator cuff. An orthopedist specializing in treating musicians told James that surgery might be needed, and that if he chose, he could see if physiotherapy and medication brought improvement.

He began physiotherapy with treatment focused on stretching, strengthening, and massage. The pain in James' left shoulder was constant, and increasing in spite of the anti-inflammatories. The exercise in therapy was often very uncomfortable.

He continued his concert schedule but became increasingly concerned about having to stop and cancel future dates. Shoulder range of motion was not improving and on the advice of a chiropractor he stopped the exercise program after two months.

I first saw James three and a half months after his injury. He described pain in his left shoulder as continuous with episodes when it became intense for two or three minutes. His active range of shoulder movement was limited to between 5° and 10° of external rotation.

Internal rotation, which also provoked pain, was limited to 35°. Shoulder extension was at 15° and flexion 130°. Abduction was quite painful after 55° and went to 120°, adduction 25°, and all motions caused pain toward the end-range. He played piano with his shoulder in moderate internal rotation, avoided much abduction, and was able to compensate with more trunk movement.

Palpation revealed thickening, puffiness, and acute soreness of the tendon of the long head of the biceps in its groove on the anterior humerus. I found restriction, tightness, swelling, and inflammation of the shoulder joint capsule, especially the superior part.

The supraspinatus tendon felt frayed, stringy, weak, and inflamed, particularly in the region under the end of the clavicle and acromion, where X-rays showed a bone spur. I began techniques to reduce swelling and organize the fibers of the biceps and supraspinatus tendons. (See illustration of shoulder region at the end of this case account.)

A start was made in improving limited anterior-posterior glide of the humeral head in the shoulder joint cavity and limited glide of the scapula over the posterior ribs. I also started Counterstrain techniques for the anterior upper thoracic spine, approached from the front of the body. Counterstrain also addressed restrictions of the left thoracic out-let, especially the lower cervical spine.

We discussed the possibility of James taking time off from his con-cert schedule. His pattern was to play the piano up to six hours daily, including practice time. He cut back practice time, but decided to con-tinue concerts for a while and then reassess. Another tour was about to begin. I showed him some very moderate shoulder exercises. His sec-ond treatment was six weeks later, after his tour.

At that second session, his condition was fairly similar to the first, with slight improvement of shoulder extension and external rotation. There was a little less inflammation and less disorganized fiber align-ment of the biceps and supraspinatus tendons. I resumed techniques to benefit the condition of the tendon tissues. Fascial Release methods focused on all the rotator cuff muscles. Treatment was also directed to the sternoclovicular joints, subclavius muscle, and suspensory liga-ment of the pleural dome. The upper ribs had many restrictions that needed attention.

James went on tour again and the third session was a month later. Active shoulder extension was now at 40°, external rotation 25°, and adduction 30°. He no longer had sharp pain episodes and the shoulder pain was no longer continuous. He was taking NSAIDs only occasion-ally after the second session and stopped entirely after the third. I con-tinued techniques to strengthen, thicken, and weave together the supraspinatus tendon. Clearing of waste products and deposits was done for this tendon as well as that of the biceps long head. The supe-rior gleno-humeral ligament portion of the shoulder joint capsule was treated for tightness and restriction.

The third treatment included further techniques to improve nar-rowing of the suprahumeral space in order to relieve an impinge-ment pattern in the shoulder. The increased space relieved excess pressure on the enclosed supraspinatus and biceps tendons. Ligament work on the joint capsule and Joint Gliding methods helped to increase mobility of the localized shoulder joint structures. Anterior-posterior glide of the humeral head had improved markedly.

James now experienced more freedom of motion and comfort in his piano playing. His range of flexion movement after the fourth session was 160°, extension at 40°, and external rotation 25°. The fourth, fifth, and sixth treatments were at three-week intervals. The left abdominal area and thorax still needed Visceral Manipulation techniques to normalize mobility of the pleura, stomach, small intestine, splenic flexure, and descending colon. Inflammation was now reduced appreciably, and mostly concentrated at the supraspinatus and biceps tendons.

At those three (fourth, fifth, sixth) treatments, I addressed elbow and wrist joint imbalances with Joint Gliding, Counterstrain, Fascial Release, and ligament work. There was more attention to the tight subscapularis muscle to allow better external rotation of the shoulder, now at 30° and still the most limited direction.

After the fourth session, at my suggestion, James began physiotherapy exercise treatment incorporating Pilates methods. He was now ready for more strengthening and stretching. He was consistent in following an exercise program using therabands while on tour. At the sixth session his shoulder flexion was at 170° and pain free, within 5° of his right side. In general he experienced slight pain only when fatigued, or at end-points of some ranges of motion (e.g., internal rotation).

With extended concert tours through Asia and Eastern Europe, James' next treatments were at six-week intervals. At the seventh session, focus was directed to continued improvement of the biceps long head tendon in its groove on the anterior humerus and attachment to the scapula. The tendon and its sheath still had slight thickening, fiber disorganization, and irritation. This condition resolved in the next three sessions.

With further attention the supraspinatus tendon continued to regain better substance, thickness, and structural organization. I worked on keeping excess waste material from accumulating in the tissue, and its frayed fiber endings were knitting together well as soreness disappeared.

At each session techniques were used for improving the openness of the suprahumeral space to allow free joint motion and reduce impingement of the soft tissues. Joint Gliding, ligament work, and Counterstrain were a benefit for shoulder joint tracking, mobility, and health of the joint capsule.

Work in the thoracic and cervical spine and joints with the ribs was resolving the compensations from James' shoulder injury with continued activity of piano playing. At the tenth session from the start of treatment his left shoulder range of motion was at normal levels. A life of piano playing has resulted in reduced external rotation of both shoulders (about 55° with the elbow bent). I saw James six months later and he was continuing to follow his busy practice and touring schedule with full comfort.

**Figure 23B**
Shoulder joint, Acromioclavicular joint.

## 13. Conoid, Trapezoid Ligaments, AC Joint Dislocation

This case can be of interest for its combination of obstacles involved, repeated setbacks, and eventual results. Daniel R. is a 59-year-old professor and former department chair at a leading university. He heads the national professional organization in his specialty. A vigorous, stocky man, he had sustained a shoulder injury in a bicycle accident three months before contacting me. The fall onto his right shoulder resulted in substantial dislocation of the acromioclavicular joint.

Daniel consulted an orthopedic surgeon well known as a shoulder specialist who diagnosed a Grade 3 AC joint dislocation with serious damage to the coracoclavicular (conoid and trapezoid) ligaments (see Figure 23B). The orthopedist felt that the ligaments could never regain functionality and that there was no good solution to the joint dislocation, with surgery having a poor prognosis.

Along with a brief course of physiotherapy, Daniel had massage and craniosacral therapy. He also began treatment with a chiropractor who applied taping to the AC joint area in an attempt at stabilization. Finding little result, she suggested a "Sully" (neoprene) brace that extended around the rib cage with strapping over the AC area. The brace provided more stability than the taping, but failed to improve the AC joint distortion or the condition of the ligaments in the two-and-a-half months he wore it continuously before I saw him.

When I first saw Daniel, the vertical discrepancy (dislocation) between the distal end of his clavicle and acromion of the scapula was larger than the width of the clavicle. I began treatment to free restrictions in the anterior shoulder joint capsule and subscapularis muscle that were pulling the head of the humerus into internal rotation. It was a major project to reposition the shoulder girdle and upper thorax in order to work on the coracoclavicular ligaments and AC joint in more normal positioning. Cushions, wedges, and some steady inferior-wards pressure on the clavicle were helpful.

The repositioning during treatment reduced the major external stresses on the ligaments and joint so that I could have more opportunity to change their internal condition. The distal end of the clavicle had to be brought more inferior and the head of the humerus moved posterior and toward external rotation so that the acromion could move superior to evenly meet the clavicle.

The trapezoid ligament was extremely overstretched, lax, and its tissue had little strength or vitality. The part showing the most tearing was close to its insertion on the undersurface of the clavicle. The ligament provided very little resistance to anterior movement of the scapula. The conoid ligament had just slightly more integrity, providing only minor resistance to posterior scapular motion. The AC joint capsule and its ligaments were very flaccid.

Treatment was started at one- and two-week intervals in which I focused on the trapezoid and conoid ligaments that normally provide the main support for stability of the joint. Weaving together and aligning the fibers, increasing their substance, strengthening the perpendicular component, clearing waste material out of their tissue, and improving local fluid circulation were all central elements of therapy. There were specific methods for improving the electrical and magnetic pulse currents in the ligaments that were weak and disorganized. By the third session, the tissue of the two ligaments was better organized and showed better pulsation and blood flow.

At the fifth session, I felt noticeably improved continuity of the trapezoid, in internal zones where it had sustained much tearing. It still needed better strength. When Daniel was supine, the alignment of the AC joint was quite good. I worked with the upper cervical spine and used cranial techniques for restrictions of the parietal bones and cranial base.

Daniel continued to use the Sully brace and receive chiropractic care for his spine. He showed admirable patience and persistence in following a therapy and exercise program. He wore the brace to stabilize the joint for many months even though it could be cumbersome. However these positive factors for his treatment were sometimes counterbalanced by his very demanding work and writing schedule, in which he continued to use the computer daily for up to eight hours, along with other work tasks. He is sometimes so absorbed in his writing and thought process that he moves in a stressful way for his shoulder.

Daniel is an avid hiker and this activity occasionally led to the other major drawback to improvement. After two months of treatment with noticeable progress he fell during a hike, destabilizing the AC joint and the ligaments. In all, several falls during the course of treatment were substantial setbacks for his shoulder.

At the session following the hiking fall, I continued to work with the spine at C6 to T1. Counterstrain and Joint Gliding were used for the upper ribs and thoracic spine. Restrictions of the tissue of the upper pleura were treated to minimize fascial pulls on Daniel's shoulder. He began to include some weights, mostly while lying down, in his home exercise program. Previously he had used only his own body weight for resistance in exercising.

Ligament work, recoil, and Fascial Release techniques were helpful for contracted tissues in the anterior right shoulder. I focused on strains in Daniel's right elbow and wrist and a structural pattern pulling his forearm into pronation. All sessions featured techniques for the ligaments. The trapezoid, which had been the weakest, was gradually regaining elasticity, substance, and firmer resistance. Four months from the start of treatment the AC joint showed good alignment when Daniel was upright at the beginning of a session.

Daniel now sometimes used a loose sling for arm support, and an elbow rest on his chair to counteract inferior pulls on the scapula while he sat the computer. In part because the pull of gravity tended to increase the discrepancy in the AC joint by pulling the head of the humerus and acromion inferior, Daniel continued to wear the brace most of the time. At four and a half months into treatment his AC joint was congruent much more of the time. At this point he had another fall, again destabilizing the joint and ligaments.

Again working to reverse a setback, I focused on the conoid ligament. This one had already improved substantially from the start of treatment. Now, after this last fall, techniques were directed to knitting together and increasing substance of the most injured part of the conoid near its lower attachment (to the coracoid process of the scapula). Working with electrical activity in the ligament to strengthen and balance its flow of current was quite useful here and in all phases of ligament treatment in this case. The trapezoid was again regaining better condition.

Daniel was able to increase intensity of his strengthening exercises. Using dumbbells in supine, 45° incline, and side lying positions, his exercise rebuilt strength in the arm, rotator cuff, chest, and back muscles. Another fall at six months into treatment again reversed some of the progress. This cycle of improvement and setbacks continued until nine months into treatment. The setbacks never reversed all progress and Daniel's condition always improved to a better level after each one.

After nine months from the start of treatment, Daniel's AC joint was almost completely congruent on a consistent basis. At this point his condition stabilized and has remained stable for six months. He stopped use of the "Sully" brace soon after the joint was consistently congruent. As the joint needed less support, the chiropractor helped him with taping to support stability. Timing of treatments went to two- or three-week intervals.

With mostly normal AC joint alignment it became possible to work more effectively with its joint capsule and its ligaments. I focused on activating, re-organizing and strengthening the tissue and fibers, which were badly over-stretched, flaccid, and weak. The capsule and its ligaments have strengthened considerably, although not to the level of the conoid and trapezoid, which have received more attention as the major support of the AC joint.

Daniel has continued to increase exercise intensity for pectoral and shoulder muscle strength. Increased muscle mass is another factor bringing his right shoulder close to a level of stability comparable to the left. Fifteen months from starting treatment, the right conoid and trapezoid ligament have for six months consistently remained only about 5% to 10% longer than those on the left. The two ligaments are still gaining steadily in substance and are now within 10% of the left side. Therapy is at four to six weeks to maintain progress as he is now quite close to full activity.

He tapes the AC joint area for more vigorous activities. Daniel is using his right arm normally for daily activities, still with some caution in heavy lifting. The condition and movement of his shoulder (gleno-humeral) joint is healthy. A setback from marathon computer use in a poor set-up while traveling caused only a brief reversal, and the AC area recovered quickly.

Daniel's course of therapy is relatively long, in response to a number of obstacles, including the setbacks. However it is quite unusual for the AC joint to regain normal congruency after such a large disloca-tion, and for the conoid and trapezoid to normalize so well after start-ing from this level of tearing and laxity.

## 14. PATELLAR LIGAMENT (TENDON)

Greg D. is a 28-year-old engineer and basketball player. He played guard on his college team, then in a summer league, and until recent-ly in weekend games at a local park. Two years before I saw him, he began to experience pain in the front of his left knee. He got shoe orthotics from a podiatrist, which provided some help for a while, but the pain increased again. The knee was most sore on landing from jumps and during backpedaling. He took NSAIDs for a while with lim-ited effect.

Greg consulted an orthopedist who diagnosed sprain of his patel-lar ligament (sometimes called patellar tendon), a condition called jumper's knee. At his suggestion Greg started physiotherapy which decreased the knee soreness for a while, but it again began to worsen. The orthopedist suggested treatment with an electrical contraction machine, but this had little effect. An MRI showed swelling and thinning of the ligament, with some evidence of tearing. At this point the orthopedist advised him to continue his exercise program and offered the option of surgery to repair and strengthen the ligament.

Greg had both chiropractic and acupuncture treatment for his knee. Both had the effect of reducing pain for a day or two, but no longer. He was taking nutritional supplements for connective tissue health. At this time he was no longer playing in basketball games, and limited to shorter periods of shooting practice with no jumping and very little running. He had increased pain climbing stairs. He became the not-so-happy owner of 25 extra pounds of increased weight that resulted from reduced activity.

Two years after knee pain started he began treatment with me. I found the patellar ligament to be swollen, weak, thin, and flaccid. Tissue wasting had apparently caused the left patellar ligament to have about 70% of the thickness of the right knee's ligament. The left patella was fixated superiorly and laterally (it was pulled up and to the lateral side). Its inferior glide was limited, putting extra pull on the ligament below it. Greg's left quadriceps muscle was tight and inflexible, especially at the distal end near the patella.

I began techniques to correct excessive inversion and fixation of the left calcaneus, which contributed to the lateral pulls on the patella. The talus and cuboid bones needed to be mobilized, as well as the ankle joint. Work was started to eliminate waste products and deposits from the ligament, and to increase its substance.

**Figure 23C**
Patellar ligament.

Quadriceps Tendon

Patella (Knee Cap)

Patellar Ligament

Tibial Tuberosity

Two weeks later, Greg told me that after the first treatment he noticed quite a different alignment through his lower leg and foot. It had at first felt odd and then he became more accustomed to it. The ligament felt better for the first three days. There was slightly less lateral pull on the patella and I worked to further reduce it by using Fascial Release methods to free restrictions of the lateral patellar retinaculum. The left knee did not extend fully, causing more strain on the patellar ligament. Joint Gliding to free the distal femur meeting with the lateral meniscus increased knee extension, as did Counterstrain for the posterior cruciate ligament. I loosened restrictions of the distal quadriceps muscle that pulled the patella upwards. The patellar ligament was a little less swollen and methods were used to organize its fiber alignment. I suggested that he continue his nutritional supplement routine.

Treatment continued at two- and three-week intervals. Greg said he noticed less pain and swelling. He was continuing stationary cycling with light resistance, and with moderate stretching and strengthening exercise from physiotherapy. I suggested he do eversion exercise with a theraband to strengthen the peroneal muscles and stabilize the lateral ankle area for better support. I showed him an additional stretch to loosen tight hamstrings that would aid knee extension. The itiotibial (IT) band at the outside of the thigh was excessively tight, as were the peroneal muscles below the knee. Fascial Release was used to loosen these structures and I suggested he also use a massage roller for the lateral thigh and lower leg soft tissues that are difficult to stretch adequately. Greg's fourth and fifth lumbar vertebrae and both sacroiliac joints needed better freedom and alignment.

At the fourth session, I continued Visceral Manipulation methods to free restrictions of the descending colon and sigmoid colon, left kidney, and small intestine that were exerting pulls down into the left leg. Techniques focused on fixations of the upper cervical spine and cranial base. The patellar ligament had better tone and felt less mushy when I worked with both the perpendicular components of its fiber for strengthening. We planned for him to use the stationary cycle for 30 minutes with more resistance.

At the fifth session I did tissue work on the pes anserinus tendons of the left knee which had been chronically sore. With more fine-tuning from Joint Gliding and Counterstrain, his knee was much closer to maintaining full joint extension. Techniques for feeding in and separating the ends of the patellar ligament were helping to increase its substance, integrity, and organization. The weakest zone was close to its inferior attachment to the top of the tibia that had sustained the most tearing. Further work with the electrical activity in the ligament was directed to increasing the circulation and vitality of its tissue. Greg said that the cycling was going well and I suggested that he do light jogging up to ten minutes on a track near his house. He also started balance training, using a rocker board.

Greg was feeling more optimistic about his knee and talked about playing basketball. We agreed that he would now jog for 15 minutes on the track and begin side-to-side stepping. I suggested he do more eccentric exercise (see Chapter 6) for his quadriceps by controlled lowering of his body in knee bends with support from his hands behind him on a counter. Techniques in the sixth treatment were directed to freeing the lateral patellar retinaculum and adjacent fascia that were still pulling the patella to the outside. I also continued methods for balancing the mobility of the anterior left hip and lumbar spine. His ankles and feet were maintaining better structural condition. The left cuboid and calcanus still needed attention to fixations.

Greg said he noticed that regular use of the roller device for massaging the quadriceps and lateral leg relieved stiffness and discomfort of his knee. In the next treatment Fascial Release was used for restrictions in the distal quadriceps and surrounding fascia connecting to the superior part of the patella. The tone of his patellar ligament was improving well and it had better perpendicular cross-linkage and thickness. I continued to work on knitting the fibers together and stimulating elasticity. We planned now for him to do 20 minutes of jogging two or three times a week. I suggested controlled lowering in knee bends on the left leg alone. He would do light basketball warm-ups in a gym and avoid jumping at this point. Playing on concrete surfaces of the park wasn't advisable.

At the eighth treatment, the focus was balancing the sacroiliac joints and freeing restrictions of the left kidney. Work with the cruciate ligaments and Joint Gliding techniques released restrictions around the lateral meniscus. This continued to establish optimal tracking of knee joint movement. Greg said that his left knee was more stable and was only slightly painful at the end of some running sessions. The pain would disappear within a few minutes or hour at the most. I suggested he do more backpedaling in his warm-ups on the court. He would do free-standing squats (knee bends) emphasizing the downward (eccentric) phase of the exercise. He would do some one-leg squats and when ready could add extra weight. He could introduce jumping and landing on two feet, but not in a game situation with contact.

With treatments at two- and three-week intervals the ninth treatment was five and a half months from the start. I worked with the internal structure of the pes anserinus (especially semitendinosus) tendons at the left knee. They were a little stiff, but no longer sore to touch. The elasticity and integrity of the left patellar ligament had improved to 80% or 90% of normal. The ligament's thickness had increased from 70% to close to 85% of the right knee ligament. Greg was starting to play basketball in light game situations without much contact for 20 minutes or one-half hour. He would only play on a wooden floor. I focused on the zone of the ligament which had originally been the most torn. The fibers of that zone were continuing to thicken and strengthen, but still needed some clearing of waste material.

Greg returned for a treatment six months later. He had continued much of his exercise program and increased some weights in resistance exercise. As athletes find it frustrating to be limited in playing their sport, he had been patient in following a treatment and conditioning program that involved a gradual return to previous activity. He had only occasional mild discomfort in his left knee, and it subsided quickly. He played basketball at the gym for up to an hour and a half, at first in light contact situations. He felt his conditioning for the sport was much better and had started to play in more serious games.

I did some fine-tuning of the knee and ankle/foot alignment. Greg's patellar ligament strength and elasticity was over 90% of normal, having been at less than 50% when treatment began. The ligament had thickened slightly since I last saw him, now to a full 85% of the right side.

### 15. Lateral Ankle Ligaments—Anterior Talo-fibular, Calcaneo-fibular

Maria C. is a 43-year-old computer technician. Since adolescence she has been involved in modern dance as a member of several performance companies. She has also been a runner for much of this time. She consulted me for chronic right ankle pain and instability.

Her ankle (distal tibia) sustained a compound fracture when she was 12. She had four major ankle sprains; the most recent was one and a half years ago. Small sprains now caused a lot of pain in the lateral ankle. Six months before I saw her, a sports/dance orthopedist said that her anterior talo-fibular ligament was hopelessly lax and the calcaneo-fibular ligament somewhat less so.

Maria had two courses of physiotherapy of about six months. Her ankle improved somewhat but the gains were not sustained. She learned some exercises from the therapy and still used them. In an effort to return to dance, she tried a course of prolotherapy injections, and an electromagnetic pulsed signal therapy in Europe, from which she found only slight benefit. She had also been receiving treatment from an osteopath. Using a taping technique for stability, she had taped her ankle constantly for four months.

When I saw Maria she was quite concerned about the ankle instability and activity limitations. She walked for exercise, avoiding uneven surfaces and hills. Her right ankle had about 6° of active dorsiflexion. The tibia was somewhat displaced anteriorly on the talus at the ankle joint. The posterior ankle ligaments were tight and shortened. Her calcaneus had an inversion pattern at the sub-talar joint, with much limitation of passive eversion. The peroneal muscles were weak in resisted active movement. The cuboid bone was fixated inferiorly.

I found her anterior talo-fibular ligament to be flaccid and almost lifeless. It was puffy and had an inert feeling. The other major lateral ankle ligament, the calcaneo-fibular, had somewhat more strength and tone, but was also quite weak and disorganized. At that first session I worked to improve mobility of the cuboid bone and to increase eversion of the calcaneus. I started to clear waste products from the lateral ligaments and increase their tone. Releasing restriction of the posterior ankle joint ligaments and Joint Gliding technique reduced the anterior displacement of the tibia on the talus at the ankle joint. When Maria got off the table to stand and walk she noticed more stability of her right lower leg and ankle.

Treatments were every four weeks and when she returned I continued many elements of the first session. Her walking was more secure. Reducing the anteriority of the tibia on the talus allowed her weight to fall more directly through the calcaneus, instead of pitching forward into the forefoot. Fascial Release and Counterstrain were used to increase calcaneal eversion.

I showed Maria a theraband exercise of calcaneal eversion to strengthen the peroneal muscles. She was to emphasize the eccentric (inward return) phase of the movement by taking four counts for the return compared to two counts for the lateral heel motion. The anterior talo-fibular ligament needed attention to a zone where the fibers were particularly disrupted and even thinner than the rest.

At the third session Maria said she had been walking on hills and feeling more stable. Her active ankle dorsiflexion was now about 10°. Her pelvis was rotated to the left and I continued methods to improve mobility of the lower trunk and spine, including Counterstrain for the anterior lower lumbars. Restrictions of the left sacroiliac and sacrococcygeal joints were lessened. Visceral Manipulation methods improved mobility of the ascending colon, cecum, right small intestine, bladder, and right kidney.

Maria reported at the fourth treatment that she now experienced ankle pain only after an hour of walking. She still used an ankle support for long walks. To improve proprioception of the ankle and foot I suggested she use a balance board with both feet initially. She continued some stretching and strengthening. Techniques to free the right cuboid bone, arch structure, subtalar and ankle joints were continued in this session. I also suggested that she regularly roll a tennis ball and handball under the arch of her foot while standing, to maintain its mobility.

Additional work with the perpendicular fiber component of the calcaneo-fibular ligament was used to further its regaining substance. Cranial, Counterstrain, and Zero Balancing methods were used to free restrictions of the upper cervical spine and cranial base.

At the fifth treatment Maria said that for the past week she had included five-minute periods of jogging in her walks. Active dorsiflexion was now at 15°. She was now ready for balance board exercise standing on one foot. I directed further attention to strengthening the anterior talo-fibular ligament. Its most weakened, torn region was now maintaining good fiber bundle alignment and gradually regaining better substance and cross-linkage.

The work included focus on the electrical activity of its tissue. These methods were promoting an increased vitality in the ligament, where it had initially seemed almost inert.

The lateral ankle area was maintaining better stability and Maria's sub-talar and ankle joints now had good balance. At the next session I worked with her posterior ankle ligaments which were becoming less fibrous and more pliable. As these posterior structures became less constricted, the habitual anteriority of the tibia at the joint needed much less attention. Maria was jogging for 15 minutes two or three times a week and planning to start dance exercise. I addressed medial left knee discomfort and habitual limitation of full joint extension. Joint Gliding and Fascial Release were used to treat the popliteus muscle and reduced mobility of the femur's articulation with the medial meniscus.

Maria started to do some dance fundamentals at home and gradually increased her running. In the seventh treatment I used Counterstrain and cranial techniques for the lumbar spine and sacroiliac joints.

Maria started attending a dance class, using caution with lateral or rotational movement and avoiding jumps. At her eighth treatment I found the anterior talo-fibular ligament to be relatively close to normal length. The ligament still did not have fully normal tone and strength although progress was substantial.

One year after that session Maria runs one-half hour regularly and attends dance classes two or three times a week. Her calcaneo-fibular ligament has good tone and normal length. The anterior talo-fibular ligament is within 10% of normal length and its stability has continued to increase. She has virtually no ankle pain.

Chapter 7 contains an overall discussion of the case accounts. The accounts are examples for the next chapter's illustration of the essential processes and tissue changes for a tendon or ligament to heal.

# Processes and Tissue Changes in Tendon/Ligament Healing —Related to Manual Therapy

**M**anual therapy can assist the essential processes and tissue changes that occur as a tendon or ligament heals from serious injury. The case studies dramatize these events. Here are the basic beneficial changes and how they may relate to my usage of targeted methods. This look at crucial processes draws a map of the primary healing factors in tendons/ligaments.

Recall that Chapter 2 contains a description of the process of chronic tendon/ligament injury. This section will illustrate how that can be reversed in the process of recovery. Examples are drawn from the primary case accounts A and B (Janet C., Robert H.). When a method is mentioned the reader may refer to the technique descriptions in Chapter 3. The assertion that the techniques can assist these favorable changes is based on research and teaching of some of the theoreticians referenced earlier, and of the clinicians developing and practicing these methods—as well as my own clinical experience.

As we see various processes and tissue changes, it is important to note that they are complementary and often interdependent.

The *reduction of excessive muscle tension* and *fascial pulls* that strain the tendon or ligament is a central process for injury healing. Robert's thumb ligament was being stressed by muscular and fascial tensions in his hand and forearm muscles. While all the techniques described in this chapter effect relaxation, the Counterstrain approach is primary for aiding the muscles' return to normal resting length. Balanced length is also assisted by work with Golgi tendon organs.

Fascial Release technique benefits tense muscles as well as normalizing the pulls through the fascial planes (including the periosteum) that tend to intersect at joints. Visceral Manipulation methods for freeing certain structures in the torso often allow the relaxation of reciprocal tension pulls through the fascias connected to the tendon or ligament. Restoration of balanced structural alignment promoted by all these methods is helpful in reducing muscular and fascial tensions. The resulting ease of the tissues improves their condition, which contributes to minimizing localized adhesions.

Methods that restore full, balanced joint motion on a proper axis (e.g., Joint Gliding technique) allow relaxation of the neighboring soft tissues, including tendons and ligaments. The soft tissues no longer need to compensate for disrupted, restricted joint motion.

A vital change is the *reduction of unhealthy cross-linkage* brought about by intermolecular bonding in problematic collagenous tissue. The clinician aims to restore good tissue metabolism and adequate mobility by reducing the adhesions and fibrosis involving: excessive misplaced cross-linkage between tendon or ligament fibers, bundles of fibers, and their interfaces with tendon sheaths and joint capsules. This was essential for Janet's fibrosed, thickened Achilles tendon and its sheath.

Healthy cross-linkage of the fibers is promoted by the restoration of optimal *inter-fiber mobility* (gliding) which is promoted by the strategy of induction that I use in Fascial Release and other osteopathic techniques (see technique descriptions in Chapter 3). Also, gently condensing the ligament enables the disorganization of the problematic fibrous binding pattern, and allows its subsequent healthy reorganization. I find this application of condensing to be congruent with the alternate feeding in and separating outward of the ends of ligaments/ tendons used in Body-Mind Centering; this also increases inter-fiber mobility and normalizes cross-linkage. Another BMC technique that is applicable here is to directly separate the fibers perpendicular to their length. Later we will see strategies for minimizing tissue inflammation, raising its metabolic rate, and increasing vascularity; all these help to reduce the "gluing" of excessive cross-linkage.

**Normal condition**

**Laxity**

**Tearing**

**Adhesions**

**Misalignment**

**Degeneration**

**Figure 24**
These basic elements of fibrous disruption were illustrated in Chapter 2's description of the injury process. This chapter will portray the reversal of these and other problems as they are changed in the recovery process.

The *restoration of normal joint mechanics* to the contiguous joint of a chronically injured tendon/ligament is a vital part of recovery, bringing major benefits for neural, circulatory, and kinesiological functions. Establishing normal mechanics includes the restoration of correct alignment, proper stability, balanced forces in the surrounding ligaments, and normal mobility of the joint. I assisted all these elements for Janet's restricted ankle joint adjacent to the injured tendon by using the methods in the next paragraph.

Counterstrain positionings treat joint dysfunctions through restoring coherent patterns of afferent input. The fulcrums of Zero Balancing, combined with its compressions and tractions, are directly aimed at normalizing joint function. Joint Gliding technique reestablishes optimal tracking of the joint on its axis and clears restrictions to full range of motion. I find that specific usage of the tissue work of Fascial Release and BMC that corrects restrictions and adhesions of the joint capsule is also beneficial for joint movement. The clinician addresses what Greenman describes as the three findings of somatic dysfunction: asymmetry, restricted motion, and tissue texture abnormality.[87]

The restoration of *adequate blood flow* and *blood/lymph drainage* in the localized injury area is important. This is vital for proper oxygenation of the area. Good fluid mechanics are promoted by reduction of excessive muscle and fascial tensions, improvement of nearby joint function, and proper alignment and mobility of the tendon/ligament fibers. I employ specific techniques for improvement of overall and localized circulatory function such as the gentle rhythmic pumping directed toward the fluid flows, which is used in BMC, and the intermittent compression and traction used in BMC and Zero Balancing.

Proper fluid drainage is instrumental for *reducing inflammation,* which is a vital part of the injury healing process. Even though her injury was no longer in the acute phase, Janet's Achilles tendon area remained swollen from inflammation and inadequate fluid drainage. Elimination of fluid accumulations (including sero-fibrinous exudate, see Chapter 2) has many benefits for reducing irritation of the tissues. Reduction of inflammation is also promoted by Counterstrain and all the other techniques I employ to reduce pressure on the tendon/ligament and adjacent areas.

Good circulation also favors the *health and abundance of the ground substance* in the ligament/tendon. This allows an increase in the ratio of its ground substance to the fibers, which is beneficial for tissue mobility and proper metabolism. This production of ground substance is stimulated by movement (after immobilization of an injury) such as intermittent tractions.

The favorable condition of adequate fluidity and ductility of the ground substance ("more sol than gel") is enhanced by raising its energy level through techniques that increase its heat, pressure, and level of electromagnetic energy. Some strategies for raising local tissue energy levels are the applications of rhythmic movement and of gentle, direct pressure to the area. Robert's thumb ligament fibers had zones of stiffness and lack of resiliency around the areas of tearing. As the ground substance of the ligament became more abundant and ductile, my palpatory sense of the tissue was that it felt more resilient, bouncy, and "juicy."

*Re-establishing the normal parallel arrangement* of the tendon/ligament fibers enables efficient functioning and tissue healing. This process is favored by the reduction of excessive, misplaced cross-linkage of fibers and their bundles, by returning the injured tendon/ligament to its proper length, and by normalizing its electromagnetic condition. The injured structures in the case accounts had generalized disruption of fibrous alignment; there were specific zones where the fibers were noticeably twisted, particularly in proximity to the areas of tearing.

Rearrangement into parallel alignment is aided through encouraging what Bainbridge Cohen calls "hooking" of the fibers, wherein they assume their natural organization in relation to one another. This inherent organization is promoted when I feed in the ends of the ligament toward each other and by the induction used in cranial osteopathy and Fascial Release techniques. It is also encouraged with my usage of very careful manual stretching of the ligament, combined with induction.

This moderate stretching is a form of the passive mobilization that the researcher S.L. Woo believes will promote the *proper remodeling of injured connective tissue structures* such as tendons.[3] Local remodeling is also promoted by restoring overall balanced structural alignment. Parallel fiber arrangement and good vascular function are components of the remodeling mechanism, which incorporates the continuous reorganization process of normal tissue. Tissue remodeling demands the appropriate level of stresses for the tendon, some of which can be provided by manual tractions.

*Improvement of neural function* is vital for healing of a tendon or ligament. For the localized tendon area this includes 1) releasing pressures on the nerves, 2) reducing excessive proprioceptor activity, 3) lowering "facilitated" (hypersensitive) reflex thresholds to normal levels, and 4) establishing coherent patterns of afferent input.

Fascial Release techniques relieve restrictive pressures along the nerve pathways, thus promoting the neurotrophic flows that provide nourishment to the target tissue. Counterstrain positionings for appropriate spinal joints and for joints near the ligament reduce tissue strains and also reduce excessive proprioceptor activity by means of an approach that is localized and also directed toward the spinal areas.

Counterstrain positionings and Joint Gliding for the spine can address what Korr calls segmental dysfunction, which includes the reflex firing patterns involving a spinal segment (cord level, bone and soft tissue) and its circuits to the body's peripheral structures.[16, 88] Segmental stress in Robert's case involved the spine at the thoracic outlet area (particularly C5, C6, C7), which impacted the injured thumb ligament. The injured ligament and its neural receptors are part of this circuit, and the improvement of its receptor activity (afferent input) was enhanced by all the techniques mentioned in this chapter, some of which decrease the localized nerve irritations caused by the excess fluid pressures and biochemistry of inflammation.

Neural function is also improved through osteopathic cranial and Visceral Manipulation techniques, which reduce reciprocal tension pulls that can pressure the nerve supply to an injured ligament. This aids the ligament by allowing restoration of balanced, undisturbed nerve transmission. Cranial techniques can harmonize the localized structure with the CNS through creating synchrony in the CRI movement patterns that connect them. Cranial techniques also assist in the reduction of overall excessive sympathetic tone, which has several advantages for injury healing.

For some tendons/ligaments that have been immobilized and weakened it is beneficial to increase proprioception as part of their activation. I promote this by using the BMC technique of low-level resistance-pressure, and also through using gentle recoil techniques (rapid release). The recoil consists of the therapist moving the body part into alignment with its force pattern (the pattern of structural pulls in that area), holding it in that position, and quickly releasing his pressure.

As a connective tissue structure such as a tendon or ligament is healing it tends to shorten unless it has beneficial conditions. The problem is often found after incomplete healing, and needs to be reversed by thinning out areas of "gluing," and lengthening the structure to achieve adequate extensibility and deformability. This process is favored by reducing adhesions and scar tissue in zones of a tendon that contain excessive cross-linkage of tendon fibers and their bundles.

My palpatory sense is that these zones of adhesed, "glued" fibers feel thick, clumped-together, shortened, and inelastic. This was most pronounced in the thickened, enlarged portions of Janet's tendon and its sheath. In applying the therapeutic strategies about to be mentioned here (and detailed earlier in the techniques section) I use specific localized contact with the zone to soften, separate, and lengthen the adhesed group of fibers, and combine this with techniques to balance and integrate it with the remainder of the tendon and its surrounding tissues.

Adequate extensibility is promoted by reducing low-grade tissue inflammation (that causes fibrosis), encouraging good fluid mechanics, and a high proportion of ground substance in the tendon/ligament. Visco-elastic structures are ideally stretched (lengthened) through gradual loading while they are heated. The heating may be accomplished through manual pressures that raise tissue energy levels (this also occurs in electromagnetic normalization). Tissue heating and loading is also effected when I use Fascial Release and stretching, Zero Balancing tractions, and the BMC techniques of alternative feeding in and elongating the ends of the ligament and separating the fibers perpendicular to their length. The desired end result is a structure with good pliability and optimal length.

Therapy to reverse degenerative change (tendinosis) in a ligament or tendon involves *clearing waste materials and deposits* from its tissues. In the tendon, the practitioner finds fatty and mucoid deposits, degraded collagen, and failed healing tissue (fibrin deposits). These deposits congest the tissue and disorganize its functions and normal fiber patterns. The feel of the tendon tissue is often a mushy, low tone consistence.

All strategies for improving fluid circulation, tissue metabolism, and oxygenation are a key to clearing waste materials. Alternate feeding in ligament ends and then separating them can loosen deposits and begin to move them out. Induction techniques for the ligament along with stretching of the tissue are also indicated. To aid elimination, employ methods to reduce high levels of pressure and tension on the local structure and surroundings. Using direct contact with the zones of the ligament containing most deposits, you can gently dissolve and move them.

I often work with the perpendicular component of the fibers as an aid to clearing the ligament infrastructure and bringing more tone to hypotonic tissues. The perpendicular approach is very useful for this condition as the fibers are usually disorganized, disrupted, and weakened by the waste materials and atrophy.

An essential component of tissue healing is the *normalization and harmonizing of its electromagnetic activity*. This process involves smooth, regular magnetic pulsation and full, free movement of electrical current in the tendon and its surroundings. Manual pressure on certain acupuncture points in the injury area and in areas adjacent to it seems to promote this mechanism. The smooth flow of electricity and magnetism is facilitated when the therapist optimizes the CRI movement through the area of the injured tendon or ligament. It may also be encouraged by the generalized effect of freeing this CRI movement in the cranial area, and then through the body connecting to the injury area. The specific method that I have developed and used for promoting normalization of electromagnetic activity in a tendon or ligament is described in Chapter 3.

Some injured ligaments or tendons (or portions of them) are weak, lax, and atrophied. Their recovery process involves *increasing their tone, substance, and thickness*. I have seen this enable lax structures to regain a more normal length. Minimizing adhesions and scar tissue formation is beneficial due to this tissue's deficiency in elasticity and strength. It is helpful to reestablish proper movement capability of the injured structure both internally and in relation to its surrounding tissues; it has been found that tendon/ligament response to non-excessive intermittent forces is an increase in thickness and strength.[1] Robert's thumb ligament needed work to correct an overall weakness and laxity and localized zones of thinning and "stringiness" of the fibers. This had resulted from extensive tearing of the ligament.

Manual techniques that I use for increasing tone are the BMC methods of using one's hand on the injured structure to aid the tissue in knitting together, and feeding in the ends of the tendon or ligament toward its center. Some of my focus in the process is on the perpendicular element of the interrelation of the fibers. These techniques can effect weaving together (length-wise and width-wise), thickening, and increased tone.

The above methods for better tone and substance appear to encourage *tissue contractility* (involving the acto-myosin motor, see Chapter 2), which favors a strengthened, more highly toned tendon or ligament. I also utilize Bainbridge Cohen's approach of increasing proprioception to encourage contractility. Through achieving adequate contractility and tone the ligament can gradually regain its proper length. Counterstrain positionings and other induction-type methods are helpful for the process of stimulating, integrating, and toning a lax ligament.

Encouraging *healthy, strong cross-linkage* of fibers is vital to remodeling and recovery. Use all the remodeling methods such as mild manual traction of the tendon when it is ready. Alternate with feeding in the ends of tendon towards its center. Improve tissue oxygenation and metabolism.

Work with the perpendicular component of the fibers increases strong intra-fiber and inter-fiber bonding as it promotes their weaving together and thickening. A vital element for good cross-linkage formation is proper fiber alignment, which can be enhanced by the above methods as well as induction techniques.

The above-mentioned techniques have some shared mechanisms for increasing substance and tissue strength: a) activating and balancing the localized tissues (e.g., neurologically), done in a non-stressful manner that is crucial in that it avoids further damage; b) improving their fluid mechanics; and c) beneficially realigning both their internal components (fibers and their bonds) and the relationship to adjacent structures such as neighboring fascias.

The first chapter contains references to the enhanced healing effects of *raising the metabolic rate of chronically injured connective tissue* (and mentions factors that may promote this). This higher rate is one of the mechanisms mentioned by Studitskii as encouraging the "plastic state," which is important for tissue repair and regeneration.[50] An increased rate of tissue metabolism may be facilitated by heat generated from manual pressure and from movement.

Likely facilitative influences for increased localized metabolism are: 1) enhanced overall energy levels in the body, 2) the increase and normalization of localized electromagnetic activity, 3) adequate, healthy ground substance in the region, and 4) adequate vascular flow resulting in healthy tissue oxygenation, nutritional supply, and waste product removal. Some influences that can heighten overall body energy levels include this increased vascular flow and a more relaxed, deeper respiration.

I have noticed that structural improvements resulting from manual therapy directly benefit circulatory and respiratory function and also enable the patient to elevate exercise levels, which further promote energy-enhancing effects. Both Robert and Janet became progressively more active in a comfortable range as they improved. There seemed to be a confluence of higher overall energy levels with increased usage, tissue health, and circulatory function of the injury areas. I used Fascial Release and related techniques that free a tendon or ligament from excessive mechanical pressures and improve its circulatory activity, thus benefiting localized tissue metabolism of the injury area.

All of the four factors mentioned in the preceding paragraph (as well as heightened tissue metabolism itself) appear to encourage the *"plastic state"* of the injured structure, which enhances repair and regeneration. This state is described in Chapter 2. The neural function involved with the recovering ligament or tendon is also an important influence in creating a plastic condition.[50]

Healthy, strong nerve currents and neurotrophic supply apparently encourage a plastic condition of the tissue. Research by Becker and others shows that tissue repair capability is boosted by enhanced nerve currents, including the DC flows.[33, 101] My use of acupressure and Zero Balancing techniques that free the movement of acupuncture energy through the tendon area can be helpful, as the meridians have been found to conduct DC current[43] (see Chapter 2). Neural function can be enhanced by use of the techniques described in the discussion of its improvement earlier in this section. Heightened nerve activity that may promote the plastic state in the tendon tissue is also stimulated by manual pressures and movement for adjacent areas and contralateral areas, which cause the activation of conditioned reflexes.

This section constructs a map of the processes and tissue changes occurring in tendon/ligament recovery and shows that they are complementary and often interdependent. The final chapter lists these shifts in a further look at all the case studies. Recovery progression for the people in the studies involved each of the positive changes pictured here, facilitated by manual therapy. The interwoven functional and structural events are essential elements of healing.

# CHAPTER 6

# SELF-HELP STRATEGIES

Here are some strategies of self-help for people with a ligament or tendon injury. In cases of serious injury this is not a substitute for professional help, although it can be a good adjunct. The first section briefly outlines primary strategies. The second section of the chapter has step-by-step guidelines of exercise and rehabilitation for four stages from onset of injury to recovery. The final section has advice on prevention and recovery for sports injuries to a ligament or tendon. The strategies here combine well with the hands-on (manual) therapy approach presented in this book.

The recovery approach in this book aims for you to be able to return to your sport, job, or other activity as quickly as possible without sacrificing the long-range health of the injury area. If you have a serious injury, it helps to know your priorities. Many competitive athletes and others with a difficult problem have the highest priority to run that marathon in two weeks or get back fast to their construction activity that caused the injury. This book's approach would help a rapid return but is most clearly suited to the person whose priority is also what their condition will be in 12 months or 12 years. Will you be fully active then because the serious injury healed well? To do that you may in the near term have to moderate activity in a program leading to a full return to sports or job activity.

The primary recovery strategies are:

• If you suspect that you have a serious injury (with major tearing) of a ligament or tendon, have it assessed by a medical/rehabilitation professional. At the least this will give you some guidelines for how protective you must be in using that part of your body. An indication of possible serious injury is that the problem area feels unstable and weak.

• Try splinting devices, taping, and supports. Though often unnecessary in the chronic stage of injury, they can be very useful for the acute stage where restricting motion (e.g., a brace for a recent ankle sprain) is extremely helpful. Signs of acute inflammation are localized redness, swelling, heat, or a high degree of pain. In chronic cases supports can be beneficial for: protection of serious injuries with major fibrous rupture; unavoidable activity that is strenuous and/or repetitive; prevention of undue pressure or strain from stretching or twisting during sleep; activity when you are fatigued.

• Adequate rest is vital to recovery. You will have to limit activity for the injury area until it can be tolerated. Injured areas need more time than normal to recuperate after usage.

• When the area around the ligament or tendon is inflamed and swollen (even in a chronic case) try to minimize this excess fluid accumulation. There are varieties of anti-inflammatory enzymes, herbs, and supplements (and in more acute cases, pharmaceuticals). It is beneficial to reduce inflammation and avoid pooling of fluids by icing and elevating the area periodically.

• Salves and ointments can be helpful, especially if the injured structure is close to the skin surface. I have seen benefit from certain homeopathic and Chinese medicine preparations and prescription creams containing a NSAID. Consult a practitioner to determine if and when their use will be helpful, as it varies for individual circumstances.

• Find ways to do pain-free movement, even if it seems limited at first.

• Maintain good circulation in the tendon or ligament, which even in normal conditions does not have much blood supply. When the injury is past the acute stage, good circulation can be promoted by aerobic exercise and some of the strategies for minimizing swelling (contrast baths, frequent brief periods of gentle movement).

• Learn to improve body mechanics for usage of the local area of the tendon or ligament. Professional advice and/or self-help guides to ergonomics for good occupational usage can help you to reduce strain from poor postural and movement patterns. The right equipment (e.g., computer workstation) and body mechanics are vital to recovery from work-related, sports, and all other injuries.

• Warm up for at least five to ten minutes (e.g., walking, dancing, or a hot shower) before stretching or strengthening exercise. Ice the injury area after exercise.

• Reduce excessive muscle tension around the ligament or tendon. It is important to be able to stretch the muscles in the surrounding region while being sure to use only a mild stretch that pulls directly on the injured structure. In some cases of serious injury, no direct stretch is beneficial while fibers are torn, very weak, or lax. Stop and/or avoid stretches where you feel pain or burning located in the localized injury area. Consult with a rehabilitation professional and/or self-help guide (see sports injury section) for guidance in beneficial, non-injurious stretching and strengthening exercise.

• Use self-massage and/or hands-on therapy as an alternative route for maintaining flexibility. You can avoid direct stretch of an injured ligament/tendon while loosening neighboring muscles with pressure from the hand, a small or medium-sized ball, or a wooden or mechanical massage tool.

• Use an outside force to do passive stretch for a muscle, ligament, or tendon. An example is using your hand to bend (flex) the opposite elbow by pulling the resting forearm up toward the shoulder (see Stage 3 of next section, Figure 26). Gentle passive stretch can be less stressful than active motion.

• Try resistance exercise to strengthen the region of the injury and restore stability. It can help restore normal tone to the ligament fibers and increase muscular support from the surrounding area. For some injuries a significant level of direct resistance pressure at the injury site is well tolerated only after a substantial portion of the healing process is established. Start with a light weight and be patient. Overall body strengthening supports recovery of the localized area.

• Do cardiovascular exercise to promote tendon/ligament healing by improving overall circulation, breathing, and metabolism. It also helps these functions locally. As long as the movement doesn't strain the injury area, some form of this activity (e.g., walking, cycling, swimming) will aid your recovery. If your work or lifestyle is sedentary, frequent brief periods of gentle movement can be helpful.

• Reestablish body equilibrium and healthy nerve communication to the injury area through balance and coordination exercise.

• Maintain good nutrition. Adequate vegetable/fruit and protein intake are important components. Supplements can be very useful, e.g.. Vitamin C is essential for nourishment of collagen in ligaments and tendons.

• Sufficient hydration seems very basic but is essential for connective tissue health. Many people do not drink enough water.

• Learn to find a baseline for experiencing the area around the ligament or tendon as fully relaxed (see Stage 2 of next section).

Coming back from serious injury involves a journey, and you can learn about the ligament or tendon and capacities you have for moving toward full recovery.

# STRATEGIES FOR FOUR-STAGE PROGRESSION OF RECOVERY, EXERCISE AFTER INJURY

These strategies are general guidelines that start from the acute stage onwards and could also apply to some kinds of chronic ligament or tendon injury. Depending on levels of pain, inflammation, and capacity to function, in chronic cases you may need to start earlier or later in this progression. If you feel that you may have a serious injury, consult a physician or other health professional in this field.

Because these are general guidelines, keep in mind that individuals vary widely in their needs and the time needed to progress through the four stages. Injuries that are quite serious or already chronic will have a different recovery timeline than the average situation (even clinicians may find it challenging to estimate the stage of healing in a person with a chronic ligament or tendon problem). It may be useful for the reader to look at the phases of injury healing in the "Remodeling Process" section of Chapter 2.

The key issue during all four stages of recovery is when to move forward with your level of activity and exercise and when to stay at the same level. If necessary it can be helpful to rest the injured area for a short period and then resume exercise when ready.

## STAGE 1

Following injury, the primary focus is to reduce pain and inflammation and find ways to do pain-free movement. Rest is very important here. Rest, ice, compression and elevation (RICE) is useful at the outset. One benefit of rest at this stage is to allow your healing collagen tissue to make its new formations. NSAIDs, herbal anti-inflammatories, salves, homeopathic remedies, anti-inflammatory enzymes, and some supplements may be helpful. Bracing or taping can protect against further injury and facilitate some movements. Physical therapy modalities like ultrasound and electrical stimulation are often beneficial at this stage.

Try to reduce inflammation and swelling by icing. Elevating the injured area helps to avoid pooling of fluids. When gentle movement is tolerated, this can also reduce swelling.

"Why wasn't Humpty-Dumpty told about RICE?"

Homeopathic salves for injured connective tissue often contain arnica or ruta. Common Chinese medicine preparations are White Flower oil, Zheng Gu Shui, and Tiger Balm. The more pungent Chinese formulas do not combine well with use of homeopathic remedies and some formulas are more appropriate after inflammation is lessened. Creams containing an NSAID (e.g., Ibuprofen) can be made by some pharmacies on prescription. These creams are helpful for inflammation if your injury is close to the skin surface.

After the first few days (usually two to five), you want to establish a base. This is a baseline level of movement and activity that is non-injurious and is a starting point for recovery. At this stage certain kinds of activity may disrupt healing, so use caution. Look for ways of doing pain-free movement. This may involve bracing or support and would include movements of the injured area that avoid the end-range of its normal motion. You can try gentle movement of the area in water. It may be fine to move the injured area in some directions, while others should be very limited. If there is no direct pain-free movement of the injury area you can exercise the opposite limb or visualize the movement, both of which can aid the injury area.

Stretching the tendon or ligament area may be painful (or inadvisable due to torn fibers) and you can then limit stretching to surrounding areas and other body regions. Mild isometric exercise may be fine after a few days. Start it well below full exertion, e.g., 30-40% effort. When only very mild exercise is done, you can sometimes do it more frequently (e. g., three or four times daily).

## STAGE 2

In the second stage of your recovery after a tendon or ligament injury, pain and swelling are somewhat lessened. While ice alone is beneficial following exercise, at this stage and throughout recovery, contrast baths that alternate heat and cold are helpful to stimulate circulation, reduce swelling, and move waste material out of the tissues. Occasional NSAIDs at times of exacerbation can reduce pain and inflammation as can more consistent use of supplements and salves, which also may promote healing.

Stretching of the non-injured areas can be done throughout in most cases. Stretching of the local area is best limited to a milder level with no end-range movement. Be very cautious with direct stretch if there has been significant tearing of ligament or tendon fibers. Pain is a crucial determinant of how much to do. Avoid bouncing stretches. Stop and/or avoid stretches where you feel pain or burning located in the localized injury area. Passive stretch (done with the aid of an outside force, see Stage 3) is often less challenging to a muscle-tendon unit than active stretch.

You can stretch and strengthen more effectively and safely after doing some warm-up to increase circulation. Walking, cycling, dancing, abdominal exercise, or any non-injurious larger region/whole body activity for five or ten minutes will be a good warm-up. Local application of heat can also increase flexibility as well as prepare for activity.

Flexibility can also be gained by self-massage of surrounding areas. It can make stretching more effective. This is particularly useful when direct stretch is problematic. Massage tools such as wooden devices and small or medium-sized balls are sometimes useful, e.g., "The Stick" (can be found on-line) is particularly good for leg muscles. Your use of mild acupressure may reduce pain and improve circulation. Cardiovascular exercise is important for good circulation and metabolism in the whole body and local injury area. If it is not painful, do walking, cycling, or swimming.

**Figure 25**
Self-massage for calf muscles. Keep lower leg relaxed. Rub and press the leg on the side of the tub or other blunt, stable border. Avoid direct pressure on the injury area or back of knee joint.

For the calf muscles you can gently press and rub the fleshy part of the lower leg on the blunt edge of a bathtub, while you keep the leg relaxed and avoid rapid movement. Similar strategies can be improvised for forearm muscles using rounded or padded (with a folded towel) corners of a stable object such as a countertop. Be careful not to directly put pressure or much pull on the injury.

Symptoms of what appears to be ligament or tendon injury can sometimes be caused by a joint problem or referred pain from another area, such as the spine. This could be a cause if you are not progressing in recovery. A health professional can assess this possibility.

Strengthening at this stage can be done with short-arch range (limited range) of motion exercise without added resistance. Isometric resistance exercise could still be good at this stage. Perhaps short-arch exercise with light resistance from therabands or tubing will also be appropriate. You can often use significant levels of resistance for muscle groups in other body regions not directly affecting the injury area.

Use the criteria of pain-free exercise and lack of pain afterward to gauge your readiness. Strengthening of the trunk for core stabilization can be beneficial to a peripheral injury. Also, it is often advantageous to mobilize the periphery (e.g., toes, fingers) for help to a more centralized problem (e.g., ankle, shoulder).

Learn to find a baseline for experiencing the area around the ligament or tendon as fully relaxed. Prolonged excessive tension around an injury is very common and is an obstacle to recovery. Relaxation of the area can be enhanced by mild heat after acute inflammation subsides (sometimes in alternation with cold), exercise involving the whole body, use of imagery, baths, biofeedback, or meditation. A skilled manual (hands-on) therapy session can deeply relax the area. Once you experience this, you can monitor the area on an ongoing basis with this baseline as a comparison to sense when it is doing well or becoming overly tight. Your memory of the relaxed state is a body experience and recalling it will reduce tension.

## STAGE 3

At this stage of recovery pain is further reduced and swelling is gone or almost eliminated. You can use contrast baths to stimulate circulation and promote removal of waste products. Warm-up before activity will allow you to move with more efficiency and safety. Some **general principles** to follow throughout all four stages are:

- Consistency of exercise

- Slow, gradual increase of exercise levels (loading) as tolerated comfortably.

- Maintenance of flexibility. Preserve or increase the resting-length of adjacent muscle(s) and range of joint motions to reduce the load on the tendon or ligament.

- Pain-free exercise in general. Slight discomfort that appears at the end of resistance exercise and dissipates soon after is acceptable.

• Specificity of exercise. When you are ready for it, do exercise that specifically involves the injured structure.

• Balance between stability and flexibility. Do not sacrifice the stability of an injured structure to increase flexibility. Both are important, but must be balanced as you progress.

**Figure 26**
Passive stretch for muscles and connecctive tissue at rear of upper arm and back of elbow. Allow left forearm to remain at rest while you lift it evenly and slowly. Stretches such as this are most beneficial when applied with an element of rotation (arrow), which avoids compressing the forearm directly into the elbow joint.

In the third stage, direct stretching is helpful, although often not to the end range of the injured ligament or tendon. You can use an outside force to do passive stretch for a muscle, ligament or tendon (see Figure 26). Gentle passive stretch can be less stressful than active motion. Controlled passive motion stimulates tensile strength of the ligament by increasing its collagen content; for this purpose the motion can be passive stretch or motion in other directions. During a stretch when you have passed the range where the muscle is elongating, you are specifically stretching the tendon or ligament. Be careful. The feeling of stretching a healthy ligament or tendon is of gradual resistance with a firm but yielding quality.

As you become more active it is still important to protect the injury area from overloading. Bracing or taping during strenuous or awkward activity will reduce loading. Awkward activities may include walking in sand or on uneven surfaces, gardening, house cleaning or repair, and activity at the end of the day or when you are tired.

For chronic injuries be sure that bracing doesn't unduly restrict motion or prevent circulation if you are using it for any length of time. While supports can be very helpful, after the acute stage do not use them excessively, because prolonged immobilization causes problems.

Identifying and correcting muscle and joint imbalances also reduces loading on the ligament or tendon. It can be helpful to consult with a health professional who will evaluate your biomechanics and offer guidance for improving them. Attention to good body mechanics can include advice on having proper equipment such as good running shoes or computer workstation.

There are some good self-help guides to ergonomics that are attentive to postural alignment and materials such as furniture and workstation. Reducing strain from poor postural and habitual usage patterns is important. Good occupational usage is essential to recovery from work-related injuries. Advice from a physical or occupational therapist (e.g., a "back school") or other movement/alignment methods such as Alexander, Body-Mind Centering, or Aston-Patterning could be beneficial.

More resistance exercise can be done, but range of motion should still be somewhat limited when you use much weight. Reducing weight bearing with water exercise (or bicycling instead of running for an ankle area injury) will enable you to maintain comfort while using increased resistance. Some injuries of the shoulder and other areas will comfortably tolerate resistance exercise done lying down that would be too stressful if done upright.

Resistance exercise that emphasizes the eccentric phase of the movement cycle can help you progress more effectively. In an eccentric contraction the muscle contracts while it is lengthening. An example is gradually lowering a hand-held weight, which causes the biceps muscle to contract and lengthen at the same time. Eccentric contraction can be emphasized by lowering the weight more slowly than you lift it in the upward phase of the biceps exercise. To focus even more on eccentric contraction and reduce strain on the injury area, you can use your other hand to help lift the weight in the upward phase, and then lower the weight with the primary arm unassisted. A program featuring eccentric exercise for treating tendon injury that has gained much publicity is explained later in this chapter's section on sport injuries.

This is a good stage to start balance training (described in Stage 4) for improving coordination.

## Stage 4

This is the last stage of recovery from a tendon or ligament injury and involves return to full health or as close as is possible. All the necessary aids featured in the earlier stages may still be helpful, and in some cases are still important. These aids include heat/cold in alternation, ice after exercise, supplements, salves, herbal or enzyme anti-inflammatories, warm-up for exercise.

You will progress from limited range-of-motion exercise to full range. As healing progresses, collagen is strengthened by the proper level of exercise, but can actually be weakened by overtraining in very strenuous activity. Pain-free exercise is still a standard to follow, except for slight discomfort at the end of resistance exercise.

Stretching is a central element, as the ability of a muscle-tendon or ligament to withstand stretch is essential for prevention of injury/re-injury. Warm-up and stretching to increase flexibility are beneficial before doing resistance exercise. If your injury involves instability from overstretched ligaments, emphasize the warm-up and overall stretching rather than the direct full-range stretch of the ligament.

Resistance exercise is important for stability and will now involve more weight bearing and greater resistance. If any habitual soreness of the tendon or ligament increases that night or the next morning, you may have done too much. It is definitely too much if there is sharp pain or if additional pain remains in the injured structure twenty-four hours after resistance or any other exercise.

When muscles have habitual zones of congestion you may do well to have them worked out by manual therapy. Skilled massage, Fascial Release, Myofascial therapy, and other methods can assist in freeing the tension in these hot spots. A guiding principle here is that the closer the therapist is working to your injured ligament or tendon, the more skill, experience, and respect for damaged tissue is demanded. Manual techniques that are fine for general muscle tension may be harmful when applied to the injury zone.

More structurally-focused hands-on methods (such as those in Chapter 3) can help you by improving localized and general alignment and balanced movement.

Maintain good nutrition, including adequate vegetables/fruits and proteins and avoiding large amounts of junk food. Drink plenty of water. This is basic; you may want to utilize supplements as well. Vitamin C is essential for nourishment of collagen in ligaments and tendons. If you have mostly vegetarian sources of protein, be attentive to the need for providing adequate, balanced protein supply and other nutritional needs which can influence connective tissue health.

Slow healing of an injury can sometimes be due to metabolic imbalances. Trace mineral deficiencies, alkaline–acid imbalance, and build-up of toxins in the body are possible factors. Although I feel some of his supplementation amounts may not be necessary, there is useful information in Bucci's writings. One of his more technical books[99] has been referenced in Chapter 2, and for general readers, *Pain Free* is a book that contains helpful information. *Beyond Aspirin*[134] is a good presentation of the issues for pharmaceuticals (NSAIDs), and some herbal anti-inflammatories that seem promising.

If you haven't already done so, this is a good time to do exercise that uses the whole kinetic chain for an entire body region, such as half-squats for a leg injury. Whole kinetic chain exercise improves not only strength and endurance, but also proprioception (sensing body position and quality of movement), balance, and coordination. Good proprioception and balance are lost in injury. They are fundamental, essential elements for recovery and prevention of re-injury.

"Smith, don't you think you should do some
balance training before going back to your
slam dunks?"

A restored sense of body position is vital for you to have proper motion control with healthy muscle firing patterns. You can do motor balance training by standing with bare feet on a carpet. Stand on one foot with eyes open, then closed and with arms down, then crossed. See if you can work up to 30 seconds with eyes closed, arms crossed on chest. Do the same with slight squatting on one leg, then half-squats. Progress to standing on a balance board or piece of foam. Walk with one foot placed directly in front of the other, heel to toe, eyes open, then closed.

Use of balance/rocker boards, Feldenkrais exercise, and resistance exercise with free weights or therabands can all help to restore healthy proprioception and balance.

# SPORTS INJURY AND RECOVERY

For sports injuries to a tendon or ligament the basic principles of recovery are:

• Consistency of exercise.

• Slow, gradual increase of exercise levels as tolerated comfortably.

• Maintenance of flexibility. Preserve or increase the resting-length of neighboring muscles and range of joint motions to reduce the load on the ligament or tendon.

• Pain-free exercise in general. Slight discomfort that appears at the end of resistance exercise and dissipates soon after is acceptable.

• Balance between stability and flexibility. Do not sacrifice the stability of an injured structure to increase flexibility. Both are important and should be balanced as you progress.

Improving proprioception, coordination, and balance will aid recovery. The tendon or ligament's connection to the nervous system involving reporting and control of body position is partially lost in injury and can be improved.

## CAUSES AND RISK FACTORS FOR SPORTS INJURIES

Causes and risk factors for ligament and tendon damage are either intrinsic (internal) factors within an athlete's body or extrinsic (external) ones.

*Intrinsic factors.* Some of these conditions within the body can be corrected:

• Misalignments of the body, e.g., excessive foot pronation, patella (kneecap) laterally displaced or riding too high on the knee joint, leg length discrepancy.

• Decreased flexibility.

- Muscle weakness or imbalance. A common example is a strong hamstring muscle not balanced by a weaker quadriceps (opposite muscle).

- Overweight.

- Joint laxity.

- Preexisting diseases, conditions. Possibilities are rheumatoid arthritis, diabetes, significant osteoarthritis of a joint, previous fracture or surgery in the localized area or in an adjacent body region.

*Extrinsic factors*. These include:

- Environmental conditions such as excessive heat, cold, high wind, high altitude.

- Poor equipment

- A tennis racket strung too tight transmits excessive forces to the elbow.

- A bicycle seat that is too low puts extra strain on the front part of the knee joint.

- Inappropriate footwear, e.g., overly rigid soles or heel counters that are too loose. Long cleats may cause problems in baseball, football, or soccer by catching and creating excessive torque on the lower leg—as contrasted with a shoe that has shorter-length cleats placed closer together.

- Sudden start to training after long inactivity or for an additional sport.

- Sudden large increase in distance or mileage for cyclists, swimmers, runners.

- Poor training surfaces or asymmetric surfaces such as the sides of hills for running.

- Excessive loads on the body.

• Repeated overload in running or jumping (All the intrinsic and extrinsic factors in this section can contribute to overloading.)

• Repeated high force throwing and overhead movements in baseball, volleyball, tennis can place large loads on the rotator cuff of the shoulder.

• Training errors. They include poor technique such as "opening up" too soon in throwing motions or issues of training intensity and rate of progression, which will be covered in the following pages on "training principles."

An example of some of the combined internal and external factors that can contribute to an athletic or dance injury is damage to an Achilles tendon caused by excessive tightness of the calf muscles, very hard training surfaces, a forefoot or heel that angles too far outward or inward, overpronation, starting hill running at high intensity.

## TRAUMATIC SPORTS INJURY, TENDON RUPTURES

Studies show that the large majority of tendons that rupture already had a lot of degenerative tissue change (described in Chapter 2).[105]

Shoulder rotator cuff tendon ruptures can happen with direct falls on the shoulder or a fall on the hand or elbow and ruptures occur more readily when there are arthritic changes (bone spurs) in the shoulder joint area.

Biceps muscle long head inserts at the shoulder; ruptures of this tendon occur in weight lifters or laborers and can happen more readily if there is shoulder joint arthritis.

The Extensor Pollicis Longus muscle pulls the thumb backward; its tendon can rupture as a delayed result of a wrist fracture.

## WHEN TO RETURN TO SPORTS AFTER AN INJURY

It is often necessary to discontinue the sports activity that caused your injury, especially when it is difficult or painful to do the activity, and the pain is increasing. After rest and rehabilitation, here are some general guidelines for restarting athletics. Return times will vary as individual athletes and injuries differ widely, depending on whether you can:

- Do non-athletic and general daily activities without pain.

- Go through arm, leg, and general motions of your sport that involve the affected area without pain.

- Perform at least moderate resistance exercise of the area and full range of joint motion easily and pain-free.

- Achieve strength of the injured body part that is very close or equal to what it was pre-injury. This level of strength would be equal or very close to that of your opposite healthy body area (e.g., opposite knee or shoulder).

Return to sports is best accompanied by continuing strength, flexibility, and balance training.

## GENERAL EXERCISE GUIDELINES FOR RECOVERY

Exercise is a vital element in healing from a tendon or ligament sports injury. For an injury that doesn't require ongoing splinting, start gentle movement for the area as soon as pain and swelling are lessened. The first objectives of exercise are to (a) encourage blood flow to the ligament or tendon, (b) reduce joint stiffness, (c) prevent weakening and wasting of the area's muscles. Goals for the next level are to bring in more strengthening.

- *Phase 1*. Look for ways of doing pain-free movement. This can involve your wearing a support or taping the injured area. Reducing gravity's pull by exercise in a pool or on an incline device can also enable movement without pain. In the early phase of recovery, isometric exercise is very helpful. Keep up flexibility of the rest of your body by stretching.

- *Phase 2*. When you can move the injured area on your own, start exercises for range of motion and basic muscle tone. These movements initially will have limited range of motion with no added resistance from an outside object. Exercise done sitting or lying down can reduce gravitational pulls. Do some warm-ups before you start the specific exercises. Various rehabilitation exercises for different body regions can be found in Micheli's[135] or Garrick's[15, 136] books.

Start exercise at 10 repetitions, one to three times a day. When you can do this much easily and without pain, increase gradually up to 20 repetitions. When you can do 20 reps easily with limited range, start exercise at 10 repetitions with increased range of motion and movement of the body weight against gravity for resistance (still no added resistance from a weight or other object.) Ice the ligament or tendon after exercise. Continue cardiovascular exercise that causes no pain.

• *Phase 3.* Add more strengthening to your exercise by using small dumbbells, weight cuffs, or rubber tubing for resistance. You will have greater range of motion of the movements. Exercise at a pain-free level and up to the point where you feel slight pain at the end of the sequence. Use the same model as in Phase 2, with your start at 10 repetitions, going up to 20, and then using more weight starting at 10. Incorporate some balance, coordination training to improve body position sensing and timely postural reflexes that are partially lost in injury. Standing and half-squats on one foot, toe raises, side-to-side jumps, and standing on a balance board are excellent balance exercise for lower body recovery. Feldenkrais exercise is a whole system aimed at neuromuscular coordination.

• *Return to Sports Activity.* After Phase 3 of exercise, when your symptoms are gone, return to sports gradually. Continue conditioning with exercise for flexibility and strength. Do weight training for strengthening of the major muscle groups in the whole region/limb of the injury. Allow adequate recovery time after sports or exercise. Recovery can involve a day between your activities and/or varying the type of activity.

A physical or occupational therapist, sports trainer, or other therapist experienced in movement for injury treatment can be extremely valuable for guidance in exercise strategies. Be sure that he/she is experienced with your injury situation. The Pilates-based program, developed at St. Francis Hospital Dance Medicine Center in San Francisco/Walnut Creek, has had much success in this area. The trainers in this program are specifically focused on exercise for recovery.

## USE OF ECCENTRIC EXERCISE

Some studies on tendinitis therapy have shown good results using eccentric exercise for strength improvement and return to sport. The studies were done with runners who had Achilles tendinitis.

Eccentric exercise is decelerating, braking activity. Picture the biceps curl with a weight in your hand. Lifting the weight is the concentric phase. In it the biceps muscle shortens as it contracts to produce force until you reach the top of the movement range with your elbow bent. You then lower the weight (eccentric phase) as your biceps muscle lengthens and contracts. In this eccentric movement phase, the biceps acts to slow down the lowering of the weight. You can also use surgical tubing, stretch bands, or other kind of weight to do this kind of exercise.

Eccentric exercise is considered quite efficient, as it produces the most force in the muscle/tendon for the least amount of energy expended. It simulates many sports movements. In many sports activities, the muscle/tendon lengthens before it contracts concentrically. An example is bending the knee somewhat (quadriceps muscle lengthens in eccentric contraction phase) before jumping.

Here is a daily eccentric exercise program for Achilles tendinitis based on the methods used by Stanish, Curwin, Mandel in Canada and Alfredson et al. in Sweden:

1. First is a warm-up of five to ten minutes. Alfredson uses stationary bicycling for warm-up.

2. Stanish suggests some stretching of the muscle-tendon.

3. Do eccentric exercise for the calf muscle/Achilles tendon by standing on a platform or step and slowly lowering the heel. Do 3 sets of 10 repetitions. This should be pain-free except for some mild pain in the final set. Weight can be added by wearing a back-pack with a weight when more load is tolerated with comfort. Speed can be increased when more load is appropriate.

4. At this point some programs use stretching.

5. Ice the tendon for at least five minutes.

**FIGURE 27**

Heel Lowering. Eccentric exercise for calf muscles, Achilles tendinitis. The athlete is using both legs for raising the body weight and one leg for lowering.

In the Canadian program, athletes can continue running as long as there is no discomfort and only mild pain. This is not possible with severe injury. Pain reduction is important and the authors suggest rest, medications, and physiotherapy modalities including ultrasound and electrostimulation.

A possible drawback of this program is lack of precise measurement of the load being applied to the tendon. The authors recommend that the best guideline to prevent exercise overloading of the injury is that mild pain only appears at the end of the 30 repetitions. Pain should not be increasing during the program and it is important that it gradually diminish as you progress in the program.

This program would not be suitable for situations where there is a serious tendon injury (major tearing, major inflammation) until other forms of rehabilitation have allowed a certain amount of healing. At that point, exercise with substantial range of joint motion and weight bearing as in this program could be appropriate. Another caution would be if there is also a significant injury to a joint in the area. A medical/exercise professional can advise on your possible readiness for an eccentric exercise program.

**"That's not what I meant by eccentric exercise."**

Some eccentric exercise can be incorporated into other recovery strategies. For a biceps curl, lower the weight more slowly (e.g., 5 counts) than you raise it upwards (e.g., 2 counts). In earlier stages of recovery it can be best to do this exercise with a limited range of motion. You can do eccentric training with assistance from your opposite non-injured leg or arm in the upward/lifting phase of the movement (e.g., using your opposite leg to lift body weight upwards on the step). This type of exercise is effective and efficient for increasing stability and strength.

### PRINCIPLES OF TRAINING AND PREVENTION

In addition to promoting success in your sport, good training patterns are a large part of preventing ligament or tendon injury or avoiding a recurrence.

### *Training Principles*

• Get some good advice on your sports technique. Use of correct body mechanics is essential in everything from swimming strokes, to skating, to a golf stroke.

• Correct muscle strength imbalances. A medical expert or trainer can help you identify and address imbalances of important muscle groups such as the balance of your hamstrings and quadriceps or the front and back muscles of your shoulder.

• Continue strength, flexibility, and balance training.

• Proper equipment is a large benefit.

• Warm up before activity.

• Pain from exercise should not be increasing over time.

• Maintain cardiovascular conditioning.

• Include some eccentric exercise training to improve conditioning and strength of important muscle/tendon areas.

• Application of some force in training (but not too much) will improve ligament and tendon integrity through increased collagen production, thickness, and cross-linking.

- Avoid sudden rapid increases in intensity, duration, or distance that can excessively overload a ligament, tendon, or other structure.

## Prevention (Including Recurrences)

In addition to all the elements of training above:

- Resolve and rehabilitate previous injuries so that they don't cause new ones, e.g., an ongoing Achilles tendon problem is a big risk factor for the knee or hip area.

- Ice after activity if there is soreness.

- Do stretching and other warm-up including heat or self-massage to increase flexibility.

- Pay attention to ongoing pain in a joint, especially if increasing: it indicates a problem that needs attention.

- Therapeutic exercise or manual (hands-on) therapy can improve alignment and joint fixations. When necessary, foot orthotics can assist with certain imbalances.

- Don't focus solely on conditioning one specific body region. If you have had knee difficulties, work also with strength, flexibility of the ankle, foot, hip and low back areas, and overall body balance.

- Allow adequate recovery time after sports or exercise.

- Activity modification is a moderation of a sports activity and can include less intensity, duration, or distance. You can use this for prevention when (1) you are fatigued or under major emotional stress, (2) you are in excessive heat, cold, high winds, high altitude, or are training on very uneven or hard surfaces, (3) You resume training after long inactivity or (4) you notice pain that might indicate an injury.

## JUMPER'S KNEE: CAUSES AND RECOVERY METHODS

This look at a very common knee injury gives an example of what to do with a sports overuse condition. Jumper's Knee is a sprain of the patellar ligament (patellar tendon). The patellar ligament runs from the bottom of the kneecap (patella) to the bony prominence on the top of the shinbone (tibia) just below it. Injury is common in sports requiring a lot of jumping, like basketball and volleyball or dance, and weightlifting involving heavy squats.

Running and kicking and rapid backward movements in soccer or tennis also place large stresses on the ligament. Causes and risk factors for injury include tight, inflexible quadriceps muscles as a major problem. Weak thigh muscles will put additional strain on the patellar ligament. Another stressor is a kneecap habitually situated too high up on the knee joint. Likewise for a kneecap that is off center toward the outside of the knee or overly loose and unstable.

**Figure 28**
**Patellar ligament of the knee.**

Some other possible risk factors for this ligament are overly pronated feet, flat feet, fixation or inversion of the heel bone, improper footwear such as very stiff soles, loose heel counters, training surfaces that are too hard (e.g., concrete), previous surgery in the area, or an inflexible hip joint.

Follow the recovery and exercise guidelines in this section. Various kinds of anti-inflammatories, supplements, salves, and bracing/support can be beneficial. After the initial phase of injury, when pain and swelling are down and you can move the injured knee yourself, start exercises for range of motion and to help prevent weakening. At first this involves exercises seated or lying down and movement of the body itself without using outside objects. Do not do exercises that cause pain. Exercise only up to a level where mild pain appears.

The next phase of exercise involves moving the body against gravity for resistance. After that you can do more strengthening by using weight cuffs and rubber tubing for added resistance. Stationary cycling can be a major help to recovery. When the symptoms are gone and your strength is normal, return to sports gradually.

After you return to sports, continue conditioning for strength and flexibility of the major upper and lower leg muscles, and for knee, hip, and ankle joint flexibility. Include attention to the peroneal muscles on the outside of the calf and the iliotibial (IT) band on the outside of the length of the thigh. These outer structures of the calf and thigh usually need massage, perhaps from a roller or massage tool, as they are difficult to stretch.

Balance training, such as standing on a rocker board or piece of foam, is important for coming back from a patellar ligament injury. Make sure that your body alignment and mechanics, sports technique, and equipment are all in good order. This often means getting some guidance from a medical/sports professional.

## Tennis Elbow: Causes and Recovery Methods

Some specific elements here of training principles and prevention for a very common sports injury are for lateral epicondylitis ("tennis elbow"). Tennis elbow is an injury to the tendon of the forearm muscles that bend the wrist backward. The tendon attaches on the bony knob at the outside of the elbow. The problem is common in racket sports like badminton, racquetball, and tennis and in work with repeated gripping activities like carpentry and homemaking and some factory jobs. Some strategies to reduce strain on the tendon are:

- Keep your wrist in neutral position for activities. Avoid gripping and pulling with wrist flexed (bent forward).

- Keep up ongoing strength and flexibility training of the biceps, triceps, wrist flexor and extensor muscles, and the shoulder area.

For tennis players in particular:

- Use a lighter racket. Graphite helps to reduce impact.

- Use your forearm for control, not power. Power comes from the legs, trunk, shoulder, and turning the hips.

• Don't freeze after hitting the ball, follow through with your stroke.

• Set racket string tension so it isn't too high.

• Hit the "sweet spot" in the center of the racket.

• Use the right footwork to achieve a good approach to the ball.

• Don't use older, heavier balls and avoid or limit play on hard surfaces like grass or concrete.

• Avoid using a "leading elbow" backhand, where your elbow is ahead of the racket at time of impact, which is overly stressful to the tendon.

**FIGURE 29**
Extensor Tendon at the Elbow.

# CHAPTER 7

# CONCLUSIONS

The course of this book illustrates a new approach to tendon/ligament healing. The therapy model I've developed is shown in action for treatment in the injury cases. The reader also sees an unusual view of the nature of these connective tissue structures.

This chapter highlights the two peoples' cases reported in depth in Chapter 4. These accounts are related to tendon/ligament healing capacity, essential changes in their recovery process, and the role of manual therapy. Other major features of the book to be seen here in light of the cases include basic principles of structural health care, sports injury and recovery, and the research study of effectiveness. This chapter also has a further view of clinical efficacy that involves favorable capabilities of a therapist for success with serious injuries. Part of the concluding summary is a look at directions in this health care area.

## Discussion of the Cases, Overview

The accounts trace healing from chronic injuries of tendons and ligaments, and the role played by the structural/osteopathic manual therapy that I provided. The data used are the author's clinical notes, the patients' reports of their condition, the reports of other clinicians, and reports of MRI findings. Discussion here contains examples from the two in-depth case accounts, in Chapter 4, which contain all the essential features of the topic. Fifteen additional case reports in that chapter portray various sports and overuse issues. The 15 cases have a similar pattern to the detailed cases, and substantiate their findings. In some general instances I will refer to "all 17" or "all" cases.

Each person's account traces progress of several variables during the course of treatment. These variables are: 1) level of comfort/pain, 2) range of motion of the joint(s) adjacent to the injury, 3) capacity for function, and 4) clinical findings such as tissue quality of the tendon/ligament (resiliency, tone, stability). In each of the 17 cases the various data sources showing progression of the different variables all indicate the subjects' consistent, gradual normalization and return to healthy condition.

The two people (Janet and Robert) in the basic cases had positive and negative indicators in their potential for recovery. Their age (both in their forties) was in the middle range for healing capacity, relative to a much younger or older person. Some other major indicators were average or above, and these include: having good overall health, adequate nutrition, a relatively stable emotional pattern, and willingness to cooperative with a treatment program. However, both injuries were quite serious—with major tearing of fibers, degeneration and other tissue damage, loss of function, little responsiveness to other forms of treatment, chronic duration, and recommendation for surgery in both cases. Their prognosis for complete recovery with surgery was uncertain. Injuries of this nature are not unusual; there is a high incidence of occupational and other disability from them.

The subjects in the cases, in response to manual therapy, appeared to demonstrate properties of tendons/ligaments which are favorable for recovery from chronic injury (see Chapter 2). These properties are: 1) significant capacity for tissue contractility, 2) a continual remodeling (self-renovation) process of connective tissue that is more extensive than in the conventional model, 3) substantial innervation of tendons/ligaments and its contribution to their influential postural and movement role (this role was improved in both cases), and 4) a capacity for healing, also more pronounced than in the conventional medical model. There seemed to be an improvement in their electrical and magnetic activity; this may exemplify the property of being responsive to electromagnetism.

While both people in the in-depth accounts exhibited all the primary aspects of serious injury and the recovery process, the two have a different emphasis. Recovery for Janet's Achilles tendon is notable for reduction of very substantial thickening, adhesion, and excessive cross-linkage of its fibers. The surrounding fascias including the tendon sheath were major structural factors here with their abnormal "gluing" to the tendon. A large nodule in the tendon was gradually normalized through the manual treatment. Janet had a very painful injury, and recovery involved a decrease of hyper-reactivity of the tendon tissue. A key to restoring her range of motion was reducing fibrosity and misplaced cross-linkage, while in Robert's case the main limitation was from pain and caution about weakness.

In Robert's recovery, his chronically weak, lax, degenerated, overstretched ligament regained good tone, length, substance, and strength. This was the most striking evidence of change. I worked to normalize thinness and "stringiness" of the fibers. The thumb ligament went through a process of restoration in regions that had very substantial tearing and wasting of fibers. Overall, his was a more fragile structure than Janet's tendon, although hers had also incurred significant rupture of fibers and neural disruption. A particular challenge for Robert's progress was demanding occupational usage of his injured hand.

Similar features of the two cases were that the injured tendon and ligament needed correction for major misalignment of normal parallel fiber arrangement. In both Janet's and Robert's situation the structure had nodules, thickened areas, and swelling. I utilized methods in each case to improve stiffness and lack of resiliency of the tissue. As they progressed, structural improvement enabled increased exercise levels leading to better circulatory and respiratory function. A resulting increase of overall bodily energy levels correlated with greater usage, better metabolism, and tissue health of the injury zone. Rest, usage with balanced alignment, and appropriate exercise were important to each person's recovery. The subjects were generally cooperative in these areas.

A basic feature of my therapy approach for all 17 people (seen in detail in the two primary accounts) were techniques to specifically and directly alter the structure of the tendon/ligament, including its microstructure (e.g., fiber re-alignment). Another basic is balancing and freeing the joints around it which were the ankle, knee, and foot joints for the Achilles tendon, and the thumb, hand, and wrist joints for the thumb ligament. Also, strategies to address the cranial, spinal, and visceral structures and their associated rhythms (e.g., CRI) are part of a whole body approach; one goal of this is to remove connecting pulls on the injury area.

All the subjects noticed major improvement (to normal levels) of their function, comfort, and range of motion. They reported that this healthy condition was still present nine months to seven years after completion of treatment. Other clinicians who had treated them also noticed these improvements, as well as healthier tissue quality of the tendon/ligament, reduced inflammation, and better function of the contiguous joint.

Processes and tissue changes that occur as a tendon or ligament heals from chronic injury (and their relation to certain manual therapy methods) are described in Chapter 5. Those that I *directly observed* for the injured tendon/ligament in all case progressions were:

- Reduction of excessive muscular and fascial pulls on it

- Restoration of normal mechanics to its associated joint(s)

- Reduction of excessive, misplaced cross-linkage and adhesion of its fibers, bundles of fibers, and surrounding structures

- Improved vascular flow through the area

- Reduced inflammation

- Restoration of its normal parallel fiber arrangement

- Improved, normalized neural function (e.g., localized decrease of hyper-reactivity)

- Restoration of adequate length, deformability (pliability) and extensibility

- Clearing the tissues of internal waste material and deposits

- Proper modeling and remodeling of its tissues

- Decreased laxity—increased strength, tone, resiliency

The following processes and tissue changes for the healing tendon/ligament in the cases were inferred and/or directly observed to a somewhat lesser degree than those listed above:

- A more fluid ground substance

- Improved, normalized neural function (e.g., healthier feedback loops and neurotrophic activity)

- Improved tissue metabolism and oxygenation

- Establishment of stronger cross-linkages

- Appearance of a "plastic state" for tissue regeneration

- Better lymphatic drainage

- Normalization of electromagnetic activity

A basic bodily healing response was described in Chapter 2, a reaction to injury that may enhance the repair process of any part of the body. Recovery for the individuals featured in the case studies appeared to include all the elements of this response. Of the "processes and tissue changes" listed above, those involving tissue re-modeling, neural responses, electromagnetic activity, the "plastic state," tissue metabolism, and vascular/lymphatic function are features of the basic bodily healing mechanism which applied to connective tissue repair for the subjects. I have reported these changes in most detail for the two primary cases.

Treatment of each person's injury includes all of the osteopathic and other non-force structural methods of my therapy model for tendons and ligaments. These were described in Chapter 3. The essential principles of these techniques listed below are all seen in the treatment picture. Another common feature is a focus on interrelation of the nervous system with the musculoskeletal system. This is particularly advantageous for treatment of tendons and ligaments, which have extensive neural involvement.

While there may be other effective therapeutic strategies for healing in similar situations it certainly appears that an in-depth, comprehensive manual therapy approach could be important for good results with serious, chronic injuries. All the case study individuals had previously received other forms of manual therapy and other conservative care without success.

There are some common essential principles of the techniques in this model which are demonstrated in the case accounts.

- Normalizing force patterns and reciprocal tension pulls in the body—combined with precise attention to localized centers of dysfunction and stress.

- Harmonizing the peripheral structures (i.e. tendon/ligament) with the center of the body and CNS (through the vertebral column and cranium).

- Re-establishing movement that is balanced and unobstructed is basic to (structural) health.

- There are intrinsic movement and force patterns in the body (i.e. CRI and optimal fluid circulation). Facilitating these patterns to operate freely is beneficial.

- Encouraging self-correction in the body. This is founded on a belief in the intelligence of the body, down to its minute components. When given the opportunity it is a self-correcting organism.

- Use of small, well-targeted changes (e.g., at the foci of physiological patterns) can have a major impact when the clinician comprehends the overall structure and dynamic.

- Combination of direct and indirect approach, with extensive usage of indirect techniques, in which the therapist follows the body's structural and movement inclination.

It is important to acknowledge the potential positive influence of nutritional strategies (including dietary and herbal supplements), stress reduction, and skilled exercise therapy to promote connective tissue healing. These can be quite effective and can be useful in combination with manual therapy.

In general my approach is best suited to injured areas which are mostly accessible to direct touch, such as those in the case studies. While the progress is slower, there have also been good results with more obscured, deeply situated structures (e.g., deeply placed spinal ligaments, see Daniel B., Case 7). It is easiest when the tissues are directly palpable, however many of the techniques (Counterstrain, BMC, ligament work, Joint Gliding, Fascial Release) are also quite useful for tendons/ligaments with limited direct access, such as the supraspinatus tendon of the rotator cuff.

Timing of the sessions can be important. For this style of therapy, which aims to promote significant structural change at each session, it is beneficial to allow at least a one-week interval. Overly frequent sessions may irritate vulnerable structures and can prevent adequate integration of previous changes. Several of the people in the case accounts responded very well to treatments at three- and four-week intervals.

A positive factor influencing recovery is a good rapport between the clinician and client. This includes confidence, sense of common direction, and timely use of humor. A good (or sometimes not-so-good) joke can be quite helpful.

A summary of the research design aspect of the book (see Chapter 4) follows for readers interested in this area. The case study design is meant to measure the efficacy of my approach. There appears to be a strong correlation between usage of the manual techniques and beneficial change for all 17 subjects.

In regard to the capacity for use of this model of manual therapy to effect injury healing for tendons/ligaments, the research design is not intended to provide proof through statistical generalization (randomized sampling). However, the case reports in context do demonstrate validation of therapeutic efficacy through analytical generalization, which relates a particular set of results (recovery from injury during therapy) to a broader model (the therapeutic model I use). Along with this deductive approach the research data establishes validation through the inductive analysis approach—which starts with specific empirical observation (recovery from injury during therapy) and builds toward a general pattern.

Multiple sources of evidence have been utilized to trace a set of variables over time, leading to the same conclusion (triangulation). This is illustrated in the progression charts at the end of both primary cases. Context is established by relating my work to the most widely used approach (standard medical) and discussing clinical theory, positive/negative indicators for success in the cases, and ways to minimize the researcher's bias. A section in Chapter 3 describes the training and experience I've had for developing technical and perceptual skills utilized to apply the clinical techniques. In sum, this supports predictive value for the case study research; usage of this therapeutic model in similar cases could provide considerable assistance in recovery.

***Sports Injury.*** The case accounts illustrate use of the author's manual therapy model to aid recovery for sports injuries from running, cycling, rowing, basketball, dance, tennis, windsurfing, and skating. The guidelines on exercise, training, and prevention for athletes in the sports injury section of Chapter 6 incorporate the principles of the therapy model. These training and fitness guidelines can be important for recovery and health maintenance, and combine well with use of the hands-on treatment for tendons and ligaments. Prevention of ligament and tendon injuries would be a valuable part of any athletic or fitness training program.

# A Further View of Clinical Efficacy

What are the crucial elements of my therapy approach that can enable positive results in cases of serious and chronic injury? Although the combination of techniques that I use is unusual, there are some practitioners who utilize one or more of them without effecting this kind of result in general. The case studies involve recovery for tendons and ligaments with substantial tearing and other damage, and loss of function—ongoing problems which had previously been unresponsive to treatment.

One element that is clearly vital for success is solid technique training with intensive grounding in the manual techniques. Instruction from expert teachers, clinical experience, independent study, and teaching has furthered my knowledge of the methods.

What else enables a practitioner to effectively use these techniques for a good outcome in difficult cases? We should emphasize the importance of the therapist as instrument, not just a mechanical tool but with accurately responsive action and perception. The skill of "listening" consists of the practitioner allowing his hand to be drawn to the center of dysfunctional structural patterns in the body as a whole, and in localized regions. Application of this valuable diagnostic method is greatly enhanced by awareness training (there is some description of this in the reference to "sensing" in the personal background section). The awareness practice can be fundamental to clinical work. It aids the capacity to synchronize and center clinical focus through a state of attentive, balanced relaxation of my own body while working.

Awareness is a crucial factor in consistent application of an alert, observational focus that is important in diagnosis and in carrying out the treatment techniques. This focus involves a type of listening that is an active receptivity utilized in monitoring the patient's body. It enables effective adjustment in the course of applying a technique and fine-tuning of the treatment while in progress. During the treatment session the practitioner may perceive that a strain pattern (unbalanced pull) is coming from within the bone in the injury area. Or the force line of the strain pattern is found to be originating in one of the various specific tissue levels (such as periosteum, cartilage, and tendon sheath) that wasn't apparent at first, but is important to address. Attentiveness allows precision in tracing body patterns to locate focal centers of structural dysfunction; and precision in promoting their beneficial change which has important overall benefit including recovery from injury.

An alert observational attention enables accuracy in both diagnostic and treatment procedures. An important factor in diagnosis is attunement to the basic body rhythms of the patient, which I also use in applying the techniques. The attunement to rhythms is made possible by the capacity of listening that enables the practitioner to establish contact with the body while disturbing its function as little as possible. An example of the value of ability for a finely tuned, precise, therapeutic approach is that a large amount of the benefit of Counterstrain positioning occurs in locating the final half to quarter inch of an exact position of release for a joint. Accurate focus is also primary for structurally detailed work with the microstructure of ligaments and tendons.

I do not intend this discussion of important capabilities to sound esoteric or overly mysterious. The capacity for concentrated attention on an ongoing basis (including awareness of subtle change of structure) is vital to this therapy approach. Emphasis here is on development of the operator as instrument, not just an interchangeable mechanical part but with a clear, active perception.

This perception and action is more clinically accurate and useful when combined with a thorough knowledge of anatomy and kinesiology. An ongoing interest in anatomy has led to continuing study that has significant application in practice. Anatomical study that includes an experiential dimension (capacity to identify and sense the structures within one's own body) seems to further enhance therapeutic efficacy. Familiarity with the body through movement derived from participation in sports, dance, and physical work (this includes the work of my clinical practice) has been very instructive and helpful in dealing with the area of a patient's physical functioning.

Another element involving personal experience that has been very useful in treating complicated cases is my own recovery from the serious, chronic tendon injury described in the "background" section of Chapter 3. The experience of finding a way to recover has deepened knowledge, insight, and confidence. It has strengthened a long-term belief in the plasticity of the body. This attitude that the body and its tissues are dynamic and responsive is a motivation to be persistent in finding strategies to improve a condition even when it is ingrained. Patience and persistence in clinical problem-solving is central.

Practicing since 1973 has given me an opportunity to thoroughly learn and experiment with different therapies and to determine if and when each is appropriate. Longevity of experience allows an advantage of seeing many different clinical situations and responses to treatment, including the emotional aspect; this is another key element of reaching good results in difficult injury cases.

## Concluding Summary: Directions in This Health Field

The approach I've developed is a therapy model for tendon/ligament healing. The model is a synthesis of various manual techniques with a particular way of applying them involving capacities of the therapist (featured in the preceding section on "efficacy"). People in the book's cases received its treatment for a variety of sports, accident, and overuse conditions.

A major goal of this book is to demonstrate how subtle and complex structural therapy can be done in a systematic, anatomically focused way. There is often a belief that subtle work is completely intuitive and without a technical, anatomical basis. I have aimed to illustrate integration of strong technical/anatomical expertise with perceptual capacity using concentrated attention, for effective clinical work.

This integration is a crucial part of my direction in this field up to the present. Readers have seen that this path also includes developing the strategies in this book for tissue and microstructure treatment of tendons and ligaments, as well as methods to incorporate their newly found physiological properties into the therapy approach. The properties involve neural response, cellular change, electromagnetism, tissue remodeling and self-repair, and contractility.

A vital future direction in this health care field is further development combining technical and perceptual skills. I am also presently exploring manual therapy strategies for cartilage injury, which is another challenging area for tissue healing. An important continuing direction that is progressing is further development of manual methods involving electricity and magnetism.

My feeling is that research on various therapeutic uses of electromagnetism for connective tissue should be of great benefit, as well as other areas of research on regeneration of tendons/ligaments. Exploring the role of satellite/stem cells in this regeneration is very intriguing. An ongoing individual focus is incorporating manual therapy with postural and exercise therapy. Increased integration of hands-on therapy with standard medicine in the health care system is also an important future direction.

The first chapter raises a variety of possibilities. My goal has been that the book's information on the topics provides a firm grounding for seeing these potentials as realistic and viable:

- Healing capacity of tendons and ligaments that is greater than seen in the standard medical model.

- Essential principles of structural health care with the body as a dynamic, responsive organism.

- Effective role of manual therapy in a new approach to sports and overuse injury.

This book's focus is a solid basis for a sense of possibility that in serious, chronic tendon and ligament injury there are avenues for a vital and natural function that is healing.

# LIST OF ILLUSTRATIONS AND PHOTOGRAPHS

# WORKS CITED IN THE TEXT

1. Levangie, P., and Norkin, C. C., *Joint Structure and Function* (F. A. Davis, Philadelphia, 2001).
2. Ganong, W., *Medical Physiology* (Appleton and Lange, Norwalk, Conn., 1992).
3. Woo, S. L.-Y, "Biomechanics of Tendons and Ligaments," *Frontiers in Biomechanics,* Woo, S. L., Schmid-Schonbein, G. W., Zweifach, B. W., eds. (Springer-Verlag, New York, 1986).
4. Kessler, R. and Hertling, D., "Assessment of Musculoskeletal Disorders," *Management of Musculoskeletal Disorders*, Kessler, R. and Hertling, D., eds. (Lippincott, Philadelphia, 1990).
5. Juhan, D., *Job's Body* (Station Hill Press, Barrytown, New York, 1987).
6. Cailliet, R., *Soft Tissue Pain and Disability* (F. A. Davis, Philadelphia, 1996).
7. Frankel, V. and Nordin, M., *Basic Biomechanics of the Skeletal System* (Lea and Febiger, Philadelphia, 1980).
8. Keene, J. S., "Ligament and Muscle-Tendon-Unit Injuries," *Orthopedic and Sports Physical Therapy*, Gould, J. and Davies, G., eds. (Mosby, St. Louis, 1985).
9. Adams, L. M., "The Anatomy of Joints Related to Function," *Mechanics of Human Joints*, Radin, E. L. and Wright, V., eds. (Dekker, New York, 1990).
10. Viidik, A., "Normal Healing of Tendons and Ligaments," *Biomechanics of Diarthrodial Joints,* Mow, V., Ratcliffe, A., Salvio, L., eds. (Springer-Verlag, New York, 1990).
11. Seedhom, B., "Ligament Reconstruction: Anterior Cruciate Ligament," *Mechanics of Human Joints,* Radin, E. L. and Wright, V., eds. (Dekker, New York, 1990).
12. Kirkaldy-Willis, W., *Managing Low Back Pain* (Churchill Livingstone, New York, 1990).
13. Paris, S. V., "The Spine" (Course Notes) (Atlanta, 1982).
14. Subotnick, S. and Sisney, P., "Treatment of Achilles Tendinopathy in the Athlete," *J Am Podiatriac Med Assoc* 76:10, 552-556 (1987).
15. Garrick, J. G. and Radetsky, P., *Anybody's Sports Medicine Book* (Ten Speed Press, Berkeley, CA, 2001).
16. Korr, I. M., *Collected Papers of I. M. Korr* (Amer. Acad. Osteopathy, Colorado Springs, 1979).

17.  Rowinski, M. J., "Afferent Neurobiology of the Joint," *Orthopedic and Sports Physical Therapy,* Gould, J. and Davies, G., eds. (Mosby, St. Louis, 1985).

18.  Lehmkuhl, L. D. and Smith, L. K., *Brunnstrom's Clinical Kinesiology* (F.A. Davis, Philadelphia, 1983).

19.  Wyke, B. D., "Articular Neurology and Manipulative Therapy," *Aspects of Manipulative Therapy,* Idczak, I. M., ed. (Lincoln Institute of Health Sciences, Victoria, Australia, 1980).

20.  Johansson, H. and Sjolander, P., "Neurophysiology of Joints," *Mechanics of Human Joints,* Radin, E. L. and Wright, V., eds. (Dekker, New York, 1990).

21.  Basmajian, J. V. and DeLuca, C., *Muscles Alive* (Williams and Wilkins, Baltimore, 1985).

22.  Radin, E. L., "Mechanically-Induced Periarticular and Neuromuscular Problems," *Mechanics of Human Joints,* Radin, E. L. and Wright, V., eds. (Dekker, New York, 1990).

23.  Bowling, R. and Rockar, P., "The Elbow Complex," *Orthopedic and Sports Physical Therapy,* Gould, J. and Davies, G., eds. (Mosby, St. Louis, 1985).

24.  LeVeau, B. F., "Basic Biomechanics in Sports and Orthopedic Physical Therapy," *Orthopedic and Sports Physical Therapy,* Gould, J. and Davies, G., eds. (Mosby, St. Louis, 1985).

25.  Kessler, R., "Friction Massage," *Management of Common Musculoskeletal Disorders,* Kessler, R. and Hertling, D. eds. (Lippincott, Philadelphia, 1990).

26.  Viidik, A. and Gottrup, F., "Mechanics of Healing Soft Tissue Wounds," *Frontiers in Biomechanics,* Woo, S. L., Schmid-Schonbein, G. W., Zweifach, B. W., eds. (Springer-Verlag, New York, 1986).

27.  Simkin, P. A., "Biology of Joints," *Mechanics of Human Joints,* Radin, E. L. and Wright, V., eds. (Dekker, New York, 1990).

28.  Jones, L. H., *Jones Strain-Counterstrain* (Jones Strain-Counterstrain Inc., Boise, ID. 1995).

29.  Hertling, D. and Kessler, R., "The Wrist and Hand Complex," *Management of Common Musculoskeletal Disorders,* Kessler, R. and Hertling, D., eds., (Lippincott, Philadelphia, 1990).

30.  Rolf, I. P., *Rolfing: The Integration of Human Structures* (Harper and Row, 1977).

31.  Korr, I. M., "Proprioceptors and Somatic Dysfunction," *J Am Osteop Assoc,* 74: 638-650 (1975).

32.  Kessler, R., "Arthrology," *Management of Common Musculoskeletal Disorders,* Kessler, R. and Hertling, D., eds., (Lippincott, Philadelphia, 1990).

33.  Becker, R. L. and Selden, G., *Body Electric* (Dekker, New York, 1990).

34.  Becker, R. L., *Cross Currents* (Putnam, New York, 1983).

35.  Becker, R. L., "Electromagnetism and Life," *Modern Bioelectricity,* Marino, A.A., ed. (Dekker, New York, 1988).

36. Marino, A., ed., *Modern Bioelectricity* (Dekker, New York, 1988).
37. Williamson, S. J., ed., *Biomagnetism: An Interdisciplinary Approach* (Plenum, New York, 1983).
38. Sisken, B., "Effects of Electromagnetic Fields on Nerve Regeneration," *Modern Bioelectricity*, Marino, A. A., ed. (Dekker, New York, 1988).
39. Smith, S., "Limb Regeneration," *Modern Bioelectricity*, Marino, A. A., ed. (Dekker, New York, 1990).
40. Gerber, R., *Vibrational Healing* (Inner Traditions, Rochester, VT, 2001).
41. Lackie, J. M., ed., *Cell Movement and Cell Behavior* (Allen and Unwin, London, 1986).
42. Hunt, V., Infinite Mind: *The Science of Human Vibrations* (Malibu, CA, 1995).
43. Reichmanis, M., "Electro-acupuncture," *Modern Bioelectricity,* Marino, A. A., ed. (Dekker, New York, 1988).
44. Abercrombie, M. and Dunn, G. A., "Locomotion and Contraction in Nonmuscle Cells," *Contractile Systems in Nonmuscle Tissues,* Perry S. V. and Margreth, A., eds. (Elsevier, Amsterdam, 1976).
45. Elzinga, M. and Lu, R., "Comparative Amino Acid Sequence Studies on Actin," *Contractile Systems in Nonmuscle Tissues,* Perry, S.V. and Margreth, A., eds. (Elsevier, Amsterdam, 1976).
46. Pollard, T. and Fujiwara, K., eds., "Participation of Contractile Proteins in Cytoplasmic Stractive and Cell Division," Perry, S. V. and Margreth, A., eds., *Contractile Systems in Nonmuscle Tissues* (Elsevier, Amsterdam, 1976).
47. Weber, K., "Biochemical Anatomy of Microfilaments of Cells in Tissue Culture," *Contractile Systems in Nonmuscle Tissues* (Elsevier, Amsterdam, 1976).
48. Strohman, R., Yamada, S., Buffinger, N., "Fibroblast Growth Factor Plays a Role in Regulating Muscle Hypertrophy," Medicine and Science in Sports and Exercise, *Am Coll Sports Med* S:173-80 (1989).
49. Strohman, R., Personal Communication (1995).
50. Studitskii, A. N., *Transplantation of Muscles in Animals* (Oxonian, New Delhi, 1988).
51. Schiaffino, S., Bormioli, S., Aloisi, M., "Fiber Branching and Formation of New Fibers During Compensatory Muscle Hypertrophy," *Muscle Regeneration*, Mauro, A., ed. (Raven, New York, 1979).
52. Carlson, B. M., "Muscle Regeneration and Aging," *Monographs in Developmental Biology* 23:189-95 (1992).
53. Moore, M. A., "Stem Cell Concepts," *Muscle Regeneration,* Mauro, A., ed. (Raven, New York, 1979).
54. Butler, D., *Mobilization of the Nervous System* (Churchill Livingstone, Melbourne, 1991).
55. Cohen, B. B., *Manuals for Courses in Body-Mind Centering* (School for Body-Mind Centering, Amherst, MA, 1977-1987).
56. Cohen, B. B., Personal Communications (1993-96).
57. Cohen, B. B., *Sensing, Feeling and Action* (Contact Editions, Northampton, MA, 1993).

58. Kessler, R. and Hertling, D., eds., *Management of Common Musculoskeletal Disorders* (Lippincott, Philadelphia, 1990).

59. Barak, T., Rosen, E., Sofer, R., "Mobility: Passive Orthopedic Manual Therapy," *Orthopedic and Sports Therapy*, Gould J. and Davies, G., eds. (Mosby, St. Louis, 1985).

60. Dyson, M., "Stimulation of Tissue Repair by Ultrasound," *Physiotherapy*, 64:105-8 (1978).

61. Forster, A., Palastanga, N., *Clayton's Electrotherapy* (Bailliere Tindall, London, 1982).

62. Palastanga, N., "Transverse Friction Massage," *Modern Manual Therapy of the Vertebral Column*, Grieve, G. P., ed. (Churchill Livingstone, Edinburgh, 1986).

63. Radin E. L., "Osteoarthrosis," *Mechanics of Human Joints*, Radin, E. L. and Wright, V. eds. (Dekker, New York, 1990).

64. Jones, L. H., Seminars, "Strain-Counterstrain" (1987, 1991).

65. College of Osteopathic Medicine of the Pacific, *Cranial Course Manual* (1985).

66. Becker, Rol., "Diagnostic Touch I and II," *Yearbooks*, Academy of Applied Osteopathy, (1963 and 1964).

67. Barral, J. P., *Visceral Manipulation* (Eastland, Seattle, 1987).

68. McPartland, J. M. and Mein, E. A., "Entrainment and the Cranial Rhythmic Impulse," *J Altern Ther Health Med* 1:40-46 (1997).

69. Smith, F. F., Seminars, "Zero Balancing" (1981-3).

70. Lippincott, H. and R., *Manual of Cranial Technique* (Edwards Brothers, Ann Arbor, 1943).

71. Magoun, H. I., *Osteopathy in the Cranial Field* (Journal Printing, Kirksville, MO, 1966).

72. Barral, J. P., *Visceral Manipulation II* (Eastland, Seattle, 1987).

73. Sutherland, W. G., *The Cranial Bowl* (Free Press, Mankato, MN, 1939).

74. Barral, J. P., *Manual Thermal Diagnosis* (Eastland, Seattle, 1996).

75. Jones, L. H., "Spontaneous Release by Positioning," *DO* 4:109-16 (1964).

76. Frymann, V. M., "A Study of the Rhythmic Motions of the Living Cranium," *J Am Osteopath Assoc* 70: 928-45 (1971).

77. Gehin, A., *Atlas of Manipulative Techniques for the Cranium and Face* (Eastland Press, Seattle, 1985).

78. Cohen, B. B., Seminar, "Fluid System," School for Body-Mind Centering (1995).

79. Barral, J. P., *The Thorax* (Eastland, Seattle, 1989).

80. Barral, J. P., *Urogenital Manipulation* (Eastland, Seattle, 1993).

81. Barral, J. P., Seminars, Visceral Manipulation (1986-93).

82. Smith, F. F., *Inner Bridges* (Humanics, Atlanta, 1990).

83. Austin M., *Acupuncture Therapy* (ASI Publishers, New York, 1972).

84. College of Osteopathic Medicine of the Pacific, *Manual of Fascial Release Techniques* (1984).

85. Becker, F., "The Meaning of Fascia and Fascial Continuity," *Osteopathic Annals* 35-47 (June, 1975).

86. Walther, D. S., *Applied Kinesiology Synopsis* (Systems D. C., Pueblo, Co., 1988).

87. Greenman, P. E., in *Neurobiologic Mechanisms in Manipulative Therapy,* Korr, I. M., ed. (Plenum, New York, 1979).

88. Patterson, M. M., in *Neurobiologic Mechanisms in Manipulative Therapy,* Korr, I. M., ed. (Plenum, New York, 1979).

89. Yin, R. K., *Case Study Research* (Sage, Thousand Oaks, CA, 1994).

90. Polkinghorne, D. E., *Phenomenological Research Methods* (Plenum, New York, 1987).

91. Nachmias, D. and Nachmias, C., *Research Methods* (Plenum, New York, 1987).

92. Patton, M. Q., *Qualitative Evaluation and Research Methods* (Sage, Newbury Park, Ca., 1990).

93. Miles, M. B. and Huberman, A. M., *Qualitative Data Analysis* (Sage, Newbury Park, Ca., 1994).

94. Merriam, S. B., *Case Study Research in Education* (Sage, Newbury Park, Ca., 1988).

95. Hoppenfeld, S., *Physical Examination of the Spine and Extremities* (Appleton-Century, Norwalk, Conn., 1976).

96. Gorman, D., *The Body Moveable* (Ampersand, Guelph, Ontario, 1981).

97. Kapandji, I. A., *Physiology of the Joints* (Churchill Livingstone, New York, 1971).

98. Helms, J. M., *Acupuncture Energetics: A Clinical Approach for Physicians* (Medical Acupuncture Publishers, Berkeley, Ca., 1995).

99. Bucci, L., *Nutrition Applied to Injury Rehabilitation and Sports Injury* (CRC Press, Boca Raton, 1995).

100. Andrews, J. R., Harrelson, G. L., and Wilk, K., *Physical Rehabilitation of the Injured Athlete* (Saunders, Philadelphia, 1998).

101. Upledger, J., and Vredevoogd, J., *Craniosacral Therapy* (Eastland Press, Seattle, 1983).

102. Stanish, W. D., Curwin, S. L., and Mandel, S., *Tendinitis: Its Etiology and Treatment* (Oxford Univ. Press, Oxford, 2000).

103. Curwin, S. L., "Tendon Injuries: Pathophysiology and Treatment," *Athletic Injuries and Rehabilitation,* Zachazewski, J. E., Magee, D. J., and Quillen, W. S., eds. (Saunders, Philadelphia, 1996).

104. El Hawary, R., Stanish, W. D., and Curwin, S. L., "Rehabilitation of Tendon Injuries in Sport," *Sports Medicine* 5:347-358 (1997).

105. Jozsa, L. G. and Kannus, P., *Human Tendons* (Human Kinetics, Champaign, IL, 1997).

106. Alfredson, H., Pietila, T., Jonsson, P. and Lorentzon, R., "Heavy-Load Eccentric Calf Muscle Training for the Treatment of Chronic Achilles Tendinosis," *Am J Sports Med* 26 (3):360-366 (1998).

107. Leadbetter, W. B., "Cell-matrix Response in Tendon Injury," *Clin Sports Med* 11 (3):533-78 (1992).

108. Huijbregts, P. A. and Smith, S. E., "Tendon Injury: A Review," *J Manual and Manipulative Therapy* 7 (2):71-80 (1999).

109. Eyre, D. R., "The Collagens of the Musculo-Skeletal Soft Tissues," *Sports-Induced Inflammation*, Leadbetter, W. B., Buckwalter, J. A., and Gordon, S. I., eds. (Am Acad Orthop Surgeons, Rosemont, IL, 1990).

110. Gehlsen, G. M., Ganion, L. R., and Helfst, R., "Fibroblast Responses to Variation in Soft Tissue Mobilization Pressure," *Med Sci Sports and Exercise* 31 (4):531-535, 1998.

111. Jain, M. K., Berg, R. A., and Tandon, G. P., "Mechanical Stress and Cellular Metabolism in Living Soft Tissue Composites," *Biomaterials* 11:465-472 (1990).

112. Almekinders, L. C. and Deol, G., "Effects of Aging, Antiinflammatory Drugs, and Ultrasound on In Vitro Response of Tendon Tissue," *Am J Sports Med* 27 (4):417-421, 1999.

113. Khan, K. M., Cook, J. L., Taunton, J. E., and Bonar, F., "Overuse Tendinosis, Not Tendinitis," *Physician and Sports Medicine* 28 (5):1-6, 2000.

114. Archambault, J. M., Wiley, J. P., and Bray, R. C., "Exercise Loading of Tendons and Development of Overuse Injuries," *Sports Medicine* 20:77-89, 1995.

115. Nirschl, R. P., "Elbow Tendinosis/Tennis Elbow," *Clinics in Sports Medicine* 11:851-870, 1992.

116. Uhthoff, H. K., Loehr, J. W., "Calcific Tendinopathy of the Rotator Cuff," *J Am Acad Orthop Surg* 5(4):183-191, 1997.

117. Wolf, W. B., "Calcific Tendinitis of the Shoulder," *Physician and Sports Medicine* 27 (9) 1-6, 2001.

118. Leadbetter, W. B., Wahl, S. M., and Barton, J., "A Possible Autoimmune Mechanism in Chronic Sports Injury," Trans 2nd Comb Meeting Orthop Research Societies, U.S.A., Japan, Europe, San Diego, CA, 391, Nov. 1995.

119. Fulcher, S. M., Kiefhaber, T. R., and Stern, P. S., "Upper Extremity Tendinitis and Overuse Syndromes in the Athlete," *Clinics in Sports Medicine* 17 (3):433-448, 1998.

120. Pedlow, P., "Focus on Eccentric Training," IDEA Personal Trainer, Sept. 2001.

121. Albert, M., *Eccentric Muscle Training* (Churchill Livingstone, London, 1995).

122. Cook, J. L., Khan, K. M., and Purdam, C., "Achilles Tendinopathy," *Manual Therapy* 7 (3):121-130, 2002.

123. Mafi, N., Lorentzon, R., and Alfredson, H., "Superior Short-term Results with Eccentric Calf Muscle Training when Compared to Concentric in a Randomized Study on Chronic Achilles Tendinosis," *Knee Surgery, Sports Traumatology* 9:42-47, 2001.

124. Silbernagel, K. G., Thomee, R., and Karlsson, J., "Eccentric Overload Training for Chronic Achilles Tendon Pain A Randomized Controlled Study," *Scand J Med Sci Sports* 11:197-206, 2001.

125. Edgelow, P., Personal Communication (2002).

126. Herold, D., Personal Communication (2002).

127. Kern-Steiner, R., Washecheck, H. S., and Kelsey, D. D., "Strategy of Exercise Using Unloading Technique for Ankle Sprain," *J Orthop and Sports Phys Ther* 29 (5):282-287, 1999.

128. Holme, E., Magnusson, S. P., "Effect of Rehabilitation on Strength, Position Sense, Re-injury Risk After Ankle Sprain," *Scand J Med Sci Sports* 9:104-109, 1999.

129. Friden, T., Roberts, D., and Zatterstrom, R., "Proprioception After Acute Knee Ligament Injury," *J Orthop Res* 15:637-644, 1997.

130. Zavatsky, A. B. and Wright, H. J., "Injury Initiation and Progression in the Anterior Cruciate Ligament," *Clinical Biomechanics* 16:47-53, 2001.

131. Loosli, A. and Oshimo, T., "Conservatively Treated Anterior Cruciate Ligament Injuries," *Clin J Sports Med* 4 (4):228-232, 1994.

132. Loosli, A. and Herold, D., "Knee Rehabilitation for Dancers Using a Pilates-based Technique," *Kinesiol and Med for Dance* 14:1-12, 1992.

133. Maagaard-Mortenson, N. H., Skov, O., and Egund, N., "Regeneration of Achilles Tendon After Necrosis," *Acta Orthop Scand* 65:87, 1994.

134. Newmark, T. M. and Schulick, P., *Beyond Aspirin* (HOHM, Prescott, AZ., 2002).

135. Micheli, L. J., *Sports Medicine Bible* (Harper, New York, 1995).

136. Garrick, J. G. and Webb, D. R., *Sports Injuries: Diagnosis and Management,* W. B. Saunders, Philadelphia, 1999).

137. Borgens, R., ed. *Electrical Fields in Vertebrate Repair* (Allen Liss, New York, 1989).

138. Greenman, P.E., *Principles of Manual Medicine* (Williams and Wilkins, Baltimore, 1996).

# BIBLIOGRAPHY

Abercrombie, M. and Dunn, G. A., "Locomotion and Contraction in Nonmuscle Cells," *Contractile Systems in Nonmuscle Tissues*, Perry S. V. and Margreth, A., eds. (Elsevier, Amsterdam, 1976).

Adams, L. M., "The Anatomy of Joints Related to Function," *Mechanics of Human Joints*, Radin, E. L. and Wright, V., eds. (Dekker, New York, 1990).

Akeson, W. H. and Frank, C. B., "Ligament Biology and Biomechanics," AAOS Symposium on Sports Medicine: The Knee, (Mosby, St. Louis 1985).

Austin M., *Acupuncture Therapy* (ASI Publishers, New York, 1972).

Barral, J. P., *Visceral Manipulation I and II* (Eastland, Seattle, 1987, 1989).

Barral, J. P., *The Thorax* (Eastland, Seattle, 1989).

Barral, J. P., *Urogenital Manipulation* (Eastland, Seattle, 1993).

Barral, J. P., *Manual Thermal Diagnosis* (Eastland, Seattle, 1996).

Basmajian, J. V. and DeLuca, C., *Muscles Alive* (Williams and Wilkins, Baltimore, 1985).

Becker, F., "The Meaning of Fascia and Fascial Continuity," *Osteopathic Annals* 35-47 (June, 1975).

Becker, R. L. and Selden, G., *Body Electric* (Dekker, New York, 1990).

Becker, R. L., *Cross Currents* (Putnam, New York, 1983).

Becker, R. L., "Electromagnetism and Life," *Modern Bioelectricity*, Marino, A.A., ed. (Dekker, New York, 1988).

Becker, R. L., "Diagnostic Touch I and II," *Yearbooks*, Academy of Applied Osteopathy (1963 and 1964).

Best, T. M. and Garrett, W. E., "Basic Science of Soft Tissue: Muscle and Tendon," *Orthopaedic Sports Medicine*, Delee, J. C. and Drez, D., eds. (W. B. Saunders, Philadelphia, 1994.)

Bogduk, N., "The Innervation of the Lumbar Spine," *Spine* 8:286-293 (1989).

Borgens, R., ed., *Electrical Fields in Vertebrate Repair* (Allen Liss, New York, 1989).

Bowling, R. and Rockar, P., "The Elbow Complex," *Orthopedic and Sports Physical Therapy*, Gould, J. and Davies, G., eds. (Mosby, St. Louis, 1985).

Butler, D., *Mobilization of the Nervous System* (Churchill Livingstone, Melbourne, 1991).

Butler, D. L., "Anterior Cruciate Ligament: Its Normal Response and Replacement," *J Orthop Res* 7: 910-921 (1989).

Cailliet, R., *Soft Tissue Pain and Disability* (F.A. Davis, Philadelphia, 1996).

Cohen, B. B., *Manuals for Courses in Body-Mind Centering* (School for Body-Mind Centering, Amherst, Mass., 1977-1987).

Cohen, B. B., *Sensing, Feeling and Action* (Contact Editions, Northampton, Mass, 1993).

Cook, J. L., Khan, K. M., and Purdam, C., "Achilles Tendinopathy," *Manual Therapy* 7 (3):121-130, 2002.

Currier, D. P. and Nelson, R. M., *Dynamics of Human Biological Tissue* (Davis, F.A., Philadelphia, 1992).

Curwin, S. L., "Tendon Injuries: Pathophysiology and Treatment," *Athletic Injuries and Rehabilitation*, Zachazewski, J. E., Magee, D. J., and Quillen, W. S., eds. (Saunders, Philadelphia, 1996).

Cyriax, J., *Textbook of Orthopedic Medicine* (Bailliere Tindall, London, 1980).

Dvorak, J. and Dvorak, V., *Manual Medicine* (Verlag, New York, 1990).

Elzinga, M. and Lu, R., "Comparative Amino Acid Sequence Studies on Actin," *Contractile Systems in Nonmuscle Tissues*, Perry, S.V. and Margreth, A., eds. (Elsevier, Amsterdam, 1976).

Farfan, H., *Mechanical Disorders of the Low Back* (Lea and Febiger, Philadelphia, 1973).

Frankel, V. and Nordin, M., *Basic Biomechanics of the Skeletal System* (Lea and Febiger, Philadelphia, 1980).

Fryette, H. H., *Principles of Osteopathic Technique* (Acad. of Applied Osteopathy, California, 1954).

Frymann, V. M., "A Study of the Rhythmic Motions of the Living Cranium," *J Am Osteopath Assoc* 70: 928-45 (1971).

Ganong, W., *Medical Physiology* (Appleton and Lange, Norwalk, Conn., 1992).

Garrick, J. and Radetsky, P., *Anybody's Sports Medicine Book* (Ten Speed Press, Berkeley, CA, 2001).

Garrick, J. G. and Webb, D. R., *Sports Injuries: Diagnosis and Management*, W. B. Saunders, Philadelphia, 1999).

Gehin, A., *Atlas of Manipulative Techniques for the Cranium and Face* (Eastland Press, Seattle, 1985).

Gerber, R., *Vibrational Healing* (Inner Traditions, Rochester, VT, 2001).

Gorman, D., *The Body Moveable* (Ampersand, Guelph, Ontario, 1981).

Gould, J. and Davies, G., eds., *Orthopedic and Sports Physical Therapy* (Mosby, St. Louis, 1985).

Greenman, P.E., *Principles of Manual Medicine* (Williams and Wilkins, Baltimore, 1996).

Grieve, G. P., ed., *Modern Manual Therapy of the Vertebral Column* (Churchill Livingstone, Edinburgh, 1986).

Guyton, A., *Textbook of Medical Physiology* (W.B. Saunders, Philadelphia, 1981).

Hoppenfeld, S., *Physical Examination of the Spine and Extremities* (Appleton-Century, Norwalk, Conn., 1976).

Hunt, T. K., Heppenstall, R. B., Pines E., eds., *Soft and Hard Tissue Repair* (Praeger, New York, 1980).

Hunt, V., *Infinite Mind: The Science of Human Vibrations* (Malibu, CA, 1995).

Johansson, H. and Sjolander, P., "Neurophysiology of Joints," *Mechanics of Human Joints*, Radin E.L. and Wright, V., eds. (Dekker, New York, 1990).

Jones, L. H., "Spontaneous Release by Positioning," *DO* 4:109-16 (1964).

Jones, L. H., *Jones Strain-Counterstrain* (Jones Strain-Counterstrain Inc., Boise, Id. 1995).

Jozsa, L. G. and Kannus, P., *Human Tendons* (Human Kinetics, Champaign, IL, 1997).

Juhan, D., *Job's Body* (Station Hill Press, Barrytown, New York, 1987).

Kapandji, I. A., *Physiology of the Joints* (Churchill Livingstone, New York, 1971).

Kessler, R. and Hertling, D., eds., *Management of Common Musculoskeletal Disorders* (Lippincott, Philadelphia, 1990).

Khan, K. M., Cook, J. L., Taunton, J. E., and Bonar, F., "Overuse Tendinosis, Not Tendinitis," *Physician and Sports Medicine* 28 (5):1-6, 2000.

Kirkaldy-Willis, W., *Managing Low Back Pain* (Churchill Livingstone, New York, 1990).

Korr, I. M., *Collected Papers of I. M. Korr* (American Academy of Osteopathy, Colorado Springs, 1979).

Korr, I. M., ed., *Neurobiologic Mechanisms in Manipulative Therapy* (Plenum, New York, 1978).

Lackie, J. M., ed., *Cell Movement and Cell Behavior* (Allen and Unwin, London, 1986).

Leadbetter, W. B., "Cell-matrix Response in Tendon Injury," *Clin Sports Med* 11 (3):533-78 (1992).

Leadbetter, W. B., Buckwalter, J. A., and Gordon, S. L., eds., *Sports-Induced Inflammation* (American Academy of Orthopedic Surgeons, Rosemont, IL, 1990).

Levangie, P. K. and Norkin, C., *Joint Structure and Function* (F.A. Davis, Philadelphia, 2001).

LeVeau, B. F., "Basic Biomechanics in Sports and Orthopedic Physical Therapy," *Orthopedic and Sports Physical Therapy*, Gould, J. and Davies, G., eds. (Mosby, St. Louis, 1985).

Lippincott, H. and R., *Manual of Cranial Technique* (Edwards Brothers, Ann Arbor, 1943).

Lundborg, G., *Nerve Injury and Repair* (Churchill Livingstone, Edinburgh, 1988).

Magee, D. J., *Orthopedic Physical Assessment* (W. B. Saunders, Philadelphia, 1997).

Magoun, H. I., *Osteopathy in the Cranial Field* (Journal Printing, Kirksville, Mo., 1966).

Marino, A., ed., *Modern Bioelectricity*, (Dekker, New York, 1988).

Mauro, A., ed., *Muscle Regeneration* (Raven, New York, 1979).

McCarty, D. J. and Koopman, W. J., eds., *Arthritis and Allied Conditions: A Textbook of Rheumatology* (Lea and Febiger, Philadelphia, 1993).

McPartland, J. M. and Mein, E. A., "Entrainment and the Cranial Rhythmic Impulse," *J Alter Ther in Health and Med* 1:40-46 (1997).

Melzack, R. and Wall, P., *Textbook of Pain* (Churchill Livingstone, Edinburgh, 1984).

Micheli, L. J., *Sports Medicine Bible* (Harper, New York, 1995).

Mow, V., Ratcliffe, A., Savio, L., eds., *Biomechanics of Diarthrodial Joints* (Springer-Verlag, New York, 1990).

Murphy, M., *The Future of the Body* (Tarcher, Los Angeles, 1992).

Nachmias, D. and Nachmias, C., *Research Methods* (Plenum, New York, 1987).

Newmark, T. M. and Schulick, P., *Beyond Aspirin* (HOHM, Prescott, AZ., 2002).

Nirschl, R. P., "Elbow Tendinosis/Tennis Elbow," *Clinics in Sports Medicine* 11:851-870, 1992.

Noyes, F. R., DeLucas, J. L., "Biomechanics of Anterior Cruciate Ligament Failure," *J Bone and Joint Surgery* 56:236-253 (1974).

Oschman, J. E. and Pert, C., *Energy Medicine: The Scientific Basis of Bioenergy Therapies* (Churchill Livingstone, New York, 2000).

Patton, M. Q., *Qualitative Evaluation and Research Methods* (Sage, Newbury Park, CA., 1990).

Perry, S.V. and Margreth, A., eds., *Contractile Systems in Nonmuscle Tissues* (Elsevier, Amsterdam, 1976).

Radin, E. L. and Wright, V., eds., *Mechanics of Human Joints* (Dekker, New York, 1990).

Radin, E. L., "Osteoarthritis," *Mechanics of Human Joints*, Radin, E. L. and Wright, V., eds. (Dekker, New York, 1990).

Reichmanis, M., "Electro-acupuncture," *Modern Bioelectricity,* Marino, A. A., ed. (Dekker, New York, 1988).

Retzlaff, E. W. and Mitchell, F. L., eds., *The Cranium and its Sutures* (Springer-Verlag, New York, 1987).

Rolf, I. P., Rolfing: *The Integration of Human Structures* (Harper and Row, 1977).

Silbernagel, K. G., Thomee, R., and Karlsson, J., "Eccentric Overload Training for Chronic Achilles Tendon Pain A Randomized Controlled Study," *Scand J Med Sci Sports* 11:197-206, 2001.

Simkin, P. A., "Biology of Joints," *Mechanics of Human Joints,* Radin, E. L. and Wright, V., eds. (Dekker, New York, 1990).

Sisken, B., "Effects of Electromagnetic Fields on Nerve Regeneration,"" *Modern Bioelectricity,* Marino, A. A., ed. (Dekker, New York, 1988).

Skalak, R. and Chien, S., *Handbook of Bioengineering* (Springer-Verlag, New York, 1987).

Smith, F. F., *Inner Bridges* (Humanics, Atlanta, 1990).

Smith, S., "Limb Regeneration," *Modern Bioelectricity,* Marino, A. A., ed. (Dekker, New York, 1990).

Stanish, W. D., Curwin, S. L., and Mandel, S., *Tendinitis: Its Etiology and Treatment* (Oxford Univ. Press, Oxford, 2000).

Stoddard, A., *Manual of Osteopathic Technique* (Hutchison, London, 1980).

Strohman, R., Yamada, S., Buffinger, N., "Fibroblast Growth Factor Plays a Role in Regulating Muscle Hypertrophy," *Medicine and Science in Sports and Exercise,* Am Coll Sports Medicine S 173-80 (1989).

Studitskii, A. N., *Transplantation of Muscles in Animals* (Oxonian, New Delhi, 1988).

Sutherland, W. G., *The Cranial Bowl* (Free Press, Mankato, Minn., 1939).

Sutherland, W. G., Sutherland, A. S., Wales, A., eds., *Collected Writings of William Garner Sutherland* (Sutherland Cranial Teaching Foundation, Kansas City, 1967).

Todd, M. E., *The Thinking Body* (Dance Horizons, New York, 1936).

Upledger, J., and Vredevoogd, J., *Craniosacral Therapy* (Eastland Press, Seattle, 1983).

Viidik, A. and Gottrup, F., "Mechanics of Healing Soft Tissue Wounds," *Frontiers in Biomechanics,* Woo, S. L., Schmid-Schonbein, G. W., Zweifach, B. W., eds. (Springer-Verlag, New York, 1986).

Viidik, A. and Vuust, J., eds., *Biology of Collagen* (Academic Press, London, 1980).

Ward, R.C., *Foundations for Osteopathic Medicine* (Lippincott, Baltimore, 1997).

Williamson, S. J., ed., *Biomagnetism: An Interdisciplinary Approach* (Plenum, New York, 1983).

Wolf, W. B., "Calcific Tendinitis of the Shoulder," *Physician and Sports Medicine* 27 (9) 1-6, 2001.

Wyke, B. D., "Neurology of the Cervical Spinal Joints," *Physiotherapy,* 65:72 (1979).

Wyke, B. D., "Articular Neurology and Manipulative Therapy," *Aspects of Manipulative Therapy*, Idczak, I. M., ed. (Lincoln Institute of Health Sciences, Victoria, Australia, 1980).

Yin, R. K., *Case Study Research* (Sage, Thousand Oaks, CA, 1994).

# ABOUT THE AUTHOR

William Weintraub has a Masters degree in Biomechanics from Antioch University. He has practiced and taught structural/osteopathic therapy in the San Francisco Bay Area for twenty-nine years. He is a Registered Movement Therapist. His extensive training in osteopathic and related methods includes Practitioner Certifications in Counterstrain technique, Body-Mind Centering, and acupressure therapy.